NURSING PHOTOBOOK™

Providing Early Mobility

NURSING83 BOOKS™
INTERMED COMMUNICATIONS, INC.
SPRINGHOUSE, PENNSYLVANIA

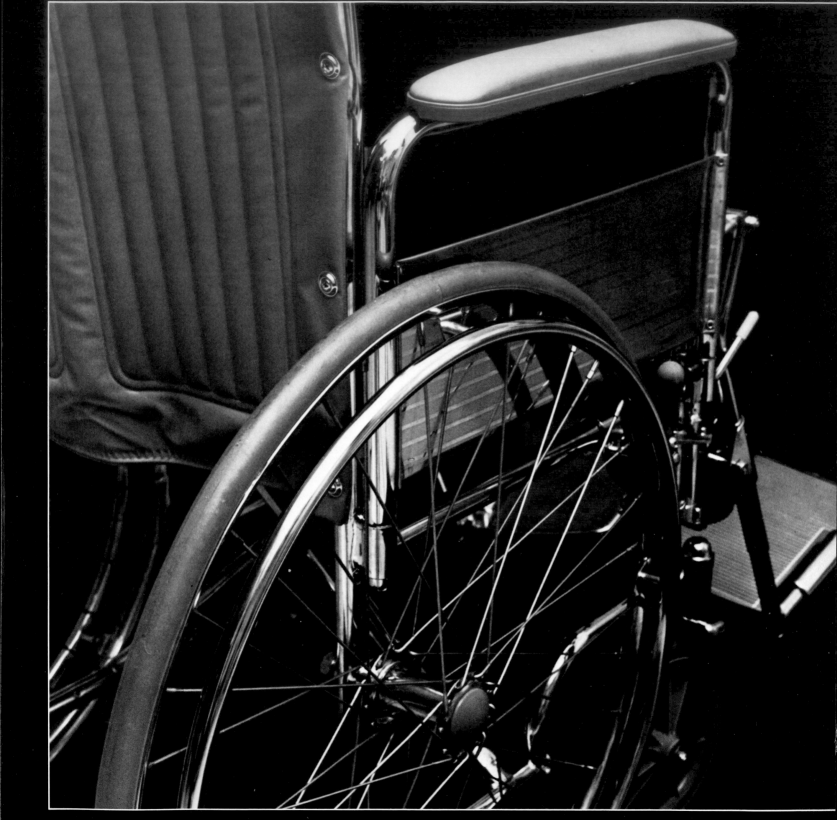

NURSING PHOTOBOOK

Providing Early Mobility

NURSING83 BOOKS™

NURSING PHOTOBOOK™ SERIES
Providing Respiratory Care
Managing I.V. Therapy
Dealing with Emergencies
Giving Medications
Assessing Your Patients
Using Monitors
Providing Early Mobility
Giving Cardiac Care
Performing GI Procedures
Implementing Urologic Procedures
Controlling Infection
Ensuring Intensive Care
Coping with Neurologic Disorders
Caring for Surgical Patients
Working with Orthopedic Patients
Nursing Pediatric Patients
Helping Geriatric Patients
Attending Ob/Gyn Patients
Aiding Ambulatory Patients
Carrying Out Special Procedures

NURSING SKILLBOOK® SERIES
Dealing with Death and Dying
Reading EKGs Correctly
Managing Diabetics Properly
Assessing Vital Functions Accurately
Helping Cancer Patients Effectively
Giving Cardiovascular Drugs Safely
Giving Emergency Care Competently
Monitoring Fluid and Electrolytes Precisely
Documenting Patient Care Responsibly
Combatting Cardiovascular Diseases Skillfully
Coping with Neurologic Problems Proficiently
Nursing Critically Ill Patients Confidently
Using Crisis Intervention Wisely

NURSE'S REFERENCE LIBRARY® SERIES
Diseases
Diagnostics
Drugs
Assessment
Procedures

Nursing83 DRUG HANDBOOK™

NURSING PHOTOBOOK™ Series
PUBLISHER
Eugene W. Jackson

EDITORIAL DIRECTOR
Jean Robinson

CLINICAL DIRECTOR
Barbara McVan, RN

ART DIRECTOR
Lisa A. Gilde

Intermed Communications
Book Division
DIRECTOR
Timothy B. King

DIRECTOR, RESEARCH
Elizabeth O'Brien

DIRECTOR, PRODUCTION AND PURCHASING
Bacil Guiley

Staff for this volume
BOOK EDITOR
Patricia Reilly Urosevich

CLINICAL EDITOR
Mary Horstman Obenrader, RN

ASSOCIATE EDITOR
Nancy Graham

PHOTOGRAPHER
Paul A. Cohen

ASSOCIATE DESIGNERS
Linda Jovinelly Franklin
Carol Stickles

CLINICAL EDITORIAL ASSOCIATE
Mary Gyetvan, RN, BSEd

EDITORIAL/GRAPHIC COORDINATOR
Doreen K. Stowers

COPY EDITORS
Barbara Hodgson
Eric R. Rinehimer

CLINICAL/GRAPHIC COORDINATOR
Evelyn M. James

ASSOCIATE PHOTOGRAPHER
Thomas Staudenmayer

EDITORIAL STAFF ASSISTANT
Cynthia A. O'Connell

DARKROOM ASSISTANTS
James M. Davidson
Gary Donnelly

ART PRODUCTION MANAGER
Wilbur D. Davidson

ARTISTS
Darcy Feralio
Diane Fox
Robert Perry
Sandra Simms
Louise Stamper
Joan Walsh
Robert Walsh
Ron Yablon

RESEARCHER
Vonda Heller

TYPOGRAPHY MANAGER
David C. Kosten

TYPOGRAPHERS
Ethel Halle
Diane Paluba

PRODUCTION MANAGER
Robert L. Dean, Jr.

ASSISTANT PRODUCTION MANAGER
Deborah C. Meiris

PRODUCTION ASSISTANT
Donald G. Knauss

ILLUSTRATORS
Gil Cohen
Jack Crane
Jack Freas
Joy Troth Friedman
Jean Gardner
Ponder Goembel
Robert Jackson
Bud Yingling

SERIES GRAPHIC DESIGNER
John C. Isely

COVER PHOTO
Seymour Mednick

Clinical consultants
for this volume
Maureen Quinn McKeown, BS, MA
Assistant Administrator of Nursing
Magee Memorial Rehabilitation Center
Philadelphia

Kathryn Nickey, BSN, MN
Associate Chief
Nursing Service for Education
VA Medical Center
Ann Arbor, Michigan

Amended reprint, 1983
© 1982, 1980 by Intermed
Communications, Inc.,
1111 Bethlehem Pike, Springhouse, Pa. 19477.
All rights reserved. Reproduction in
whole or part by any means
whatsoever without written permission
of the publisher is prohibited by law.

PB-040483

Library of Congress
Cataloging in Publication Data

Main entry under title:

Providing early mobility.

(Nursing Photobook Series)
Bibliography: p.
Includes index.
1. Transport of sick and wounded.   2. Sick—Posi-
tioning.   3. Human Mechanics.   4. Nursing.   5. Re-
habilitation nursing.   I. Title: Early mobility.
[DNLM: 1. Early ambulation—Nursing texts.   2. Re-
habilitation—Nursing texts.   WY 152 P969]
RT87.T72P76   610.73   80-25062
ISBN 0-916730-27-1

Contents

Introduction

Preparing for early mobility

CONTRIBUTORS TO
THIS SECTION INCLUDE:
Barbara J. Morgan, RPT
Virginia Sisney Sharpless, RN, AB, MSN
Marilyn Wullschleger, RN, BSN

10 Goal setting
13 Using basic body mechanics
18 Turning and positioning
46 Reviewing exercises
62 Special considerations

Performing transfer techniques

CONTRIBUTORS TO
THIS SECTION INCLUDE:
Beth Jacobs, RN
Michelle Young, RN, MS

72 Preparing for transfers
76 Performing transfers

Aiding mobility with special equipment

CONTRIBUTORS TO
THIS SECTION INCLUDE:
Barbara J. Morgan, RPT

104 Crutches, canes, and walkers
129 Wheelchairs

Dealing with special situations

CONTRIBUTORS TO
THIS SECTION INCLUDE:
Bonnie Blossom, RPT

136 Environmental considerations

153 Agencies listing
154 Home assessment form
156 Selected references
158 Acknowledgements
158 Index

Contributors

At the time of original publication, these contributors held the following positions.

Bonnie Blossom is chief physical therapist at the Center for Rehabilitation Medicine, Emory University, Atlanta, Ga. She received her BS from Washington State University in Pullman, and an MA from Georgia State University in Atlanta. She earned her physical therapy certification from the U.S. Army Medical Specialist Program. Ms. Blossom's a member of the American Physical Therapy Association.

Beth W. Jacobs is head nurse at Magee Memorial Rehabilitation Center in Philadelphia, Pa. She's a graduate of the Methodist Hospital School of Nursing, Philadelphia. In addition to being a member of the Pennsylvania Chapter of the Greater Delaware Valley District of the Association of Rehabilitation Nurses' Board of Directors, she belongs to the Association of Rehabilitation Nurses.

Maureen Quinn McKeown, one of the advisers on this book, is assistant director of nursing at Magee Memorial Rehabilitation Center, Philadelphia, Pa. A graduate of the Suffolk School of Nursing, Southampton (N.Y.) Hospital, she received her BS from Long Island University, Brooklyn, N.Y. and her MA from New York University. She's a member of the American Congress of Physical Medicine and Rehabilitation, the Pennsylvania Chapter of the Greater Delaware Valley District of the Association of Rehabilitation Nurses, the Association of Rehabilitation Nurses, and Sigma Theta Tau.

Barbara J. Morgan received her BS from the University of Kentucky in Lexington and her MEd at Colorado State University in Fort Collins. She's a physical therapist at the Rehabilitation Research and Training Center, University of Colorado Health Sciences Center, Denver. Ms. Morgan is a member of the American Physical Therapy Association.

Kathryn Nickey, also an adviser for this book, is associate chief, nursing service for education, at the VA Medical Center, Ann Arbor, Mich. A graduate of Indiana University School of Nursing, Indianapolis, she earned her BSN from the University of Tennessee (Memphis) College of Nursing and her MN from the University of Washington in Seattle. She's a member of the American Nurses Association, the Association of Rehabilitation Nurses, and Sigma Theta Tau.

Virginia Sisney Sharpless is a nursing instructor at the spinal cord injury service, VA Medical Center, Long Beach, Calif. She's a graduate of the Baptist Memorial School of Nursing, Memphis, Tenn., and received an AB degree from Union University, Jackson, Tenn., and an MSN from Emory University, Atlanta, Ga. Ms. Sharpless belongs to the Association of Rehabilitation Nurses.

Marilyn J. Wullschleger is a nursing instructor in the rehabilitation and spinal cord injury service at the VA Medical Center, Long Beach, Calif. She's a graduate of the California Lutheran Hospital School of Nursing in Los Angeles, and earned her BSN from the University of Southern California, also in Los Angeles. She belongs to the American Congress of Rehabilitation Medicine, and the Association of Rehabilitation Nurses.

Michelle Young earned her BSN from the University of Rochester (N.Y.), and her MS at Boston (Mass.) University. Ms. Young is coordinator of education at Magee Memorial Rehabilitation Center, Philadelphia, Pa. In addition, she's a member of the Association of Rehabilitation Nurses, Pennsylvania Chapter of the Greater Delaware Valley District of the Association of Rehabilitation Nurses, the Black Nurses Association, and the National Spinal Cord Injury Foundation.

Introduction

Whether you know it or not, you play an important role in helping your patient achieve early mobility. Obviously, you're not a rehabilitation expert. Nevertheless, you spend more time with your patient than any other health-care professional. And by understanding the skills required, you can help your patient make the most of his abilities, as quickly as possible.

With this in mind, we asked eight nurses and physical therapists to contribute to this NURSING PHOTOBOOK. Our objective? To assist you in taking a positive approach to the emotional and physical considerations in early mobility.

What makes *Providing Early Mobility* different from other mobility books on the market? To begin with, we've included step-by-step procedures and photos for turning and positioning, range-of-motion and isometric exercises, and transfer techniques.

We've also included the detailed instruction you need to use the following pieces of transfer and positioning equipment: cradle boots, hand rolls, footboards, hand splints, transfer boards, and mechanical lifters.

A major portion of this book focuses on the physical and emotional preparation of your patient for early mobility. In this section, you'll learn how to use a drawsheet to move a patient from a side-lying to a prone position, and how to help prepare your patient for a leg amputation. You'll be guided through the procedures for wrapping stumps—both above-the-knee and below-the-knee. You'll also find out how to improve your body mechanics to help avoid personal injury, and look and feel better.

In other sections of the book, our concise captions and how-to-do-it photos will show you how to safely transfer a patient with halo traction; how to select the proper crutches, cane, walker, or wheelchair for your patient; and how to teach him to use the equipment correctly.

But your duties don't stop here. You'll have to give continuing support and encouragement to your patient and his family. This PHOTOBOOK will offer some suggestions on how you can help your patient adapt to the environment outside the hospital. It features guidelines for recommending adaptive equipment, such as reachers, ramps, and lapboards.

As you'll see, *Providing Early Mobility* contains a wealth of information and practical nursing tips. We believe this book will help you and your patient take a positive step toward mobility.

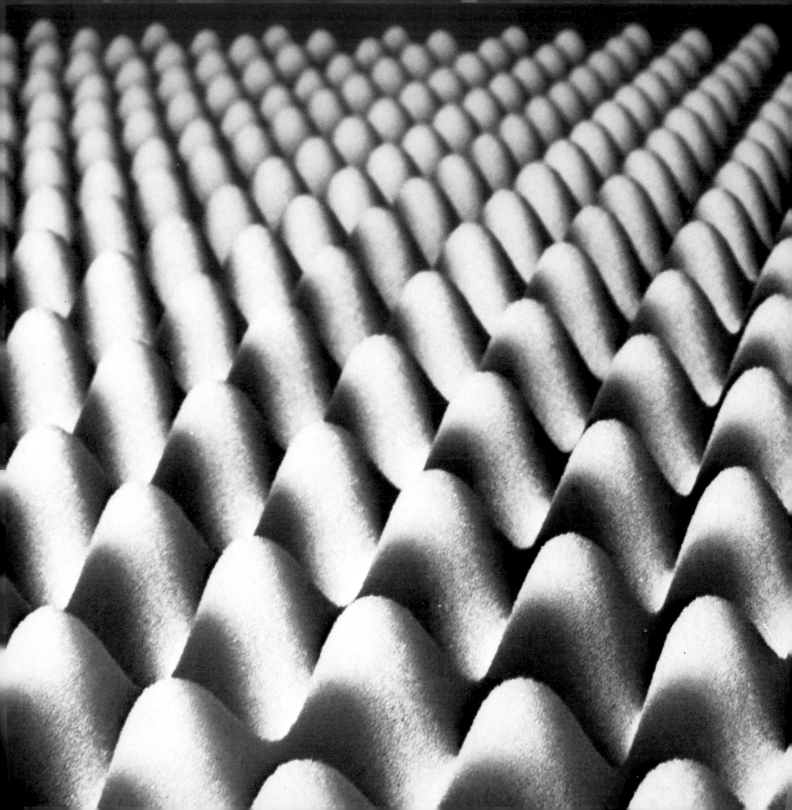

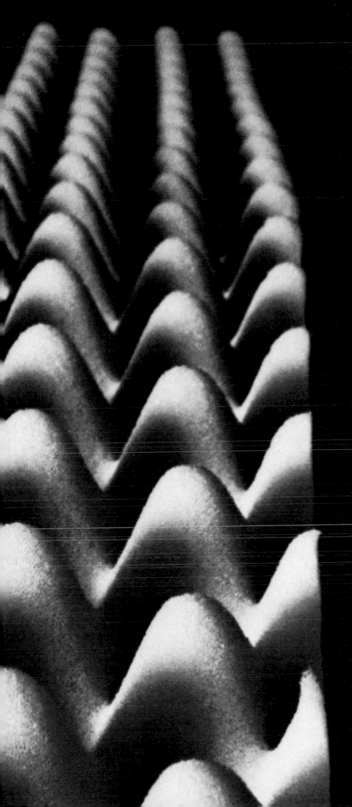

Preparing for Early Mobility

Goal setting
Using basic body mechanics
Turning and positioning
Reviewing exercises
Special considerations

Goal setting

Early mobility. Finding ways to help your patient attain it should be part of each care plan. But helping your patient adjust to his condition and work toward mobility isn't always easy. You'll have to consider his mental and physical status before you begin.

Do you know how to assess your patient's mental status? What questions to ask his family and friends? How to establish proper atmosphere for goal setting? What if your patient's angry, depressed, or tired?

How does goal setting fit into early mobility? Do you know what your role in goal setting is?

Learning as much as possible about your patient's condition is your first responsibility. To prepare yourself for this important task, study the information on the next few pages.

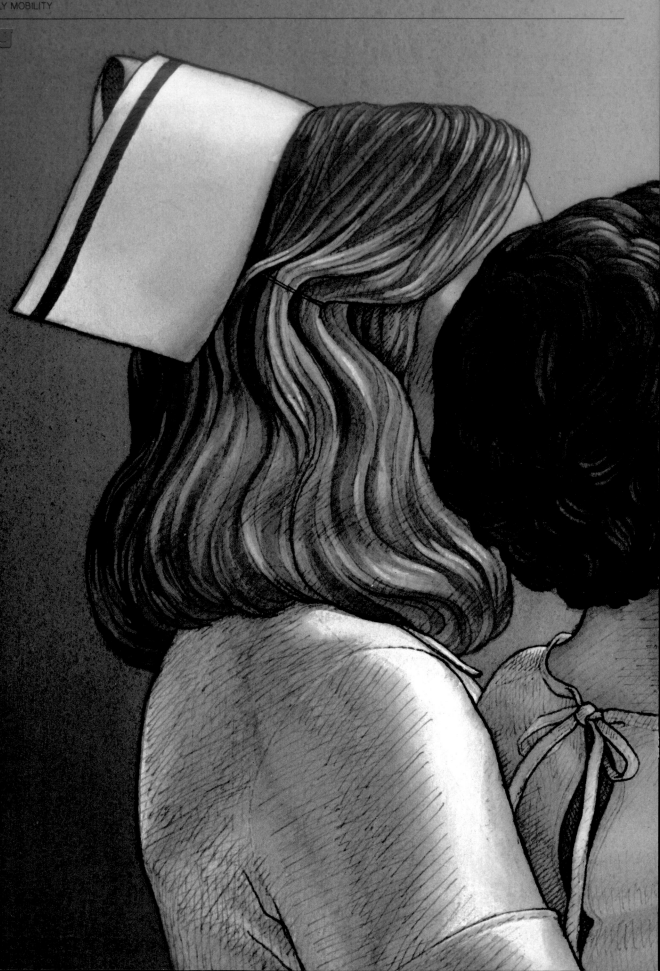

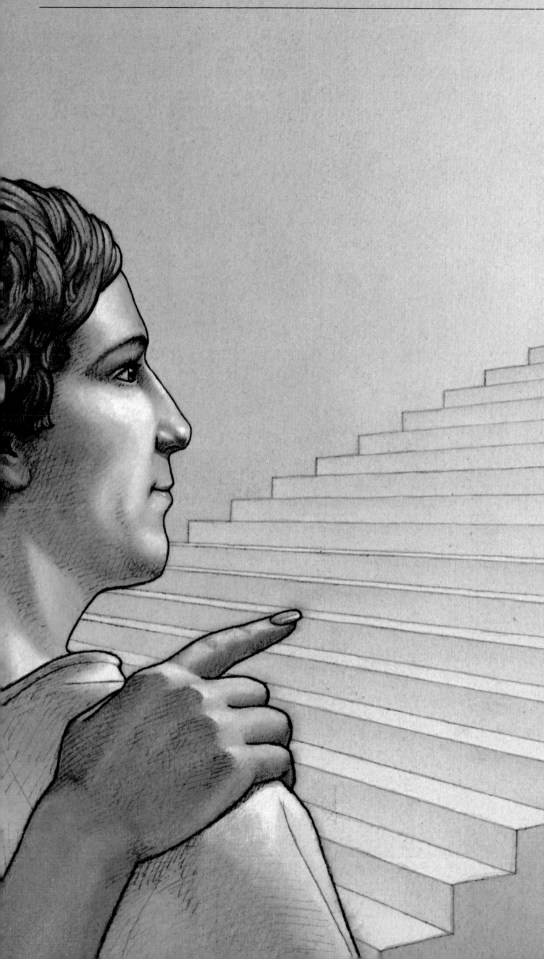

Assessing your patient's condition

Wondering how to prepare your patient for early mobility? Begin by assessing your patient's physical and mental condition, then document your findings. Here's how:

• **Observe his physical condition.** Is he in pain? Does he have weakness or paralysis of any limbs? Does he have any limb contractures or deformities? Are any limbs missing? Does he have any preexisting skin conditions? How well does he see, hear, smell, and respond to touch? Does he have a partial or total sensory deficit? How mobile is your patient? For example, can he move about in bed? Does he have any other physical limitations? If he does, are they recent? If he's had them for a while, how has he adapted to his condition (if at all)?

• **Check his care plan and medical history.** Has the doctor or physical therapist left specific instructions regarding your patient's care? Does his care plan and medical history provide you with any information on his willingness and ability to learn?

• **Evaluate your patient's mental and emotional status.** What's his level of consciousness? Is he alert and oriented? Does he appear anxious, afraid, confused, or uninterested? How's his memory? How does he react to you, his family, friends, and other health-care professionals? What's your estimate of your patient's intellectual capacity? What does he know about his condition and prognosis? Does he have a clear understanding of them? What's his attitude: one of fear, guilt, denial, or acceptance? Does he recognize his strengths and limitations? Is he willing and eager, and motivated toward greater independence?

• **Ask your patient about his goals (if he has any at this time).** Are his expectations realistic? Is it likely that he'll eventually achieve his goals? What's his attitude toward himself?

• **Talk to your patient's family and friends.** What do they know about your patient's condition and prognosis? How are they accepting his hospitalization? Can they provide you with additional information about your patient; for example, home environment, financial status, or his reactions to past illnesses? Do they seem willing and able to help your patient achieve greater independence? What are their expectations? Are these expectations realistic?

Finally, if you've done a thorough job assessing your patient, you should be able to answer the following questions: *What does my patient do for himself? What can he do for himself? What does he want to do for himself?*

When you have the answers to these questions, you can begin planning the goal-setting session.

Goal setting

Goal setting: What's your role?

Before you help your patient set long- and short-term goals, be sure you know all the facts about your patient's condition and get more information, if needed. Then, try to anticipate your patient's questions and try to answer them completely and honestly. If you're not sure how to answer, tell your patient you'll get the information for him. Show the same consideration for his family and friends, who'll also have questions.

Allow your patient time to adjust to his condition. If he's tired, agitated, or depressed, postpone your goal-setting session for a better time. Try to understand the effect his condition has on his emotions.

Remember, your patient may also feel apprehensive and upset about being hospitalized, so help him relax. Establish a rapport with him. Encourage your patient to talk about his feelings.

You'll need your patient's cooperation and confidence. If you can't successfully motivate your patient to participate in a productive goal-setting session, ask a coworker to try. As you know, motivation comes from within a patient, and each patient will adjust to his condition differently.

Here are some guidelines that will help you gain cooperation from your patient:
• Accept his condition realistically, yet with a positive outlook.
• Maintain control over your emotions.
• Encourage your patient to participate in the goal-setting session.
• Make sure his short-term goals are attainable.
• Guard against setting time limits for short- or long-term goals.

How to help your patient set short- and long-term goals

After you assess your patient mentally and physically, goal setting is the next step toward mobility. After doing a thorough assessment, you'll want to help him set realistic goals. Be sure to use good judgment when you arrange an appointment to talk with your patient. Make the time mutually agreeable. Then, before your meeting, allow him plenty of time to think and talk about goal possibilities. Suggest he include family or friends in his plans. Here's how to proceed when you begin the session:

First, make sure your patient's comfortable and that you have sufficient privacy. Then, encourage him to discuss possible long-term goals. Be certain he understands that his long-term goals should be geared toward his true capabilities, not the possibly unrealistic expectations of his family and friends.

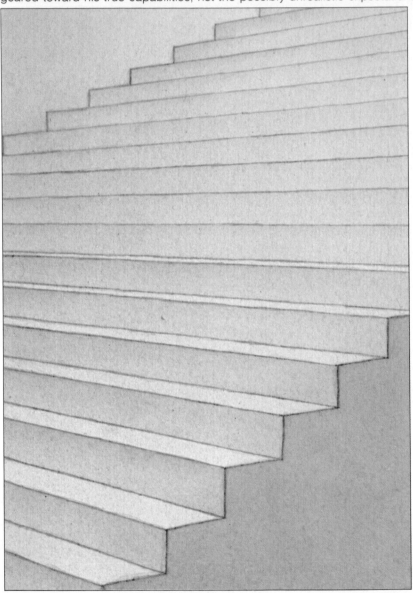

Remember: Your patient may find it easier to set only short-term goals. For example, if your patient's aphasic, he may not be able to see his potentials realistically. Later, he may feel better prepared to set long-term goals.

Suppose your patient's had a CVA, with resulting right-sided hemiplegia. In this situation, a realistic long-term goal may be to walk with a cane. But, if your patient's had a total T_6 spinal transection, such a goal would be impossible. Instead, a realistic long-term goal may be total wheelchair independence. Other long-term goals for a patient with a T_6 spinal transection may be:
• limited ambulation with long leg braces and crutches
• independent transfer to a motor vehicle
• total self-care.

After your patient decides on a realistic long-term goal, recommend he set several short-term goals, such as the following (which are appropriate to many patients):
• turning himself in bed
• dressing his upper body
• feeding himself
• helping care for himself
• transferring himself from bed to wheelchair using a transfer board with or without assistance
• improving his balance while sitting or standing
• helping others get him to and from a commode chair.

Remember, your patient's short-term goals should be attainable. Hopefully, by achieving his short-term goals, he'll gain confidence and become more motivated to achieve his long-term goal.

Important: Never set inflexible time limits for short- or long-term goals. Remember, each patient will achieve his goals at his own speed. If you set an inflexible time limit, your patient may feel unnecessarily frustrated or depressed if he fails to meet the schedule.

Another reminder: Don't forget to praise your patient for his participation in the goal-setting session.

Using basic body mechanics

Reviewing posture basics

How much do you know about body mechanics? Using basic body mechanics will help you avoid injuries, as well as look and feel better. In addition, you'll set a good example for your patient. But, do you know where to begin?

Do you know how to sit correctly? How to lift a package from a high shelf? Or how to stand properly?

The answers to these questions and others are listed on the following pages. Study them carefully.

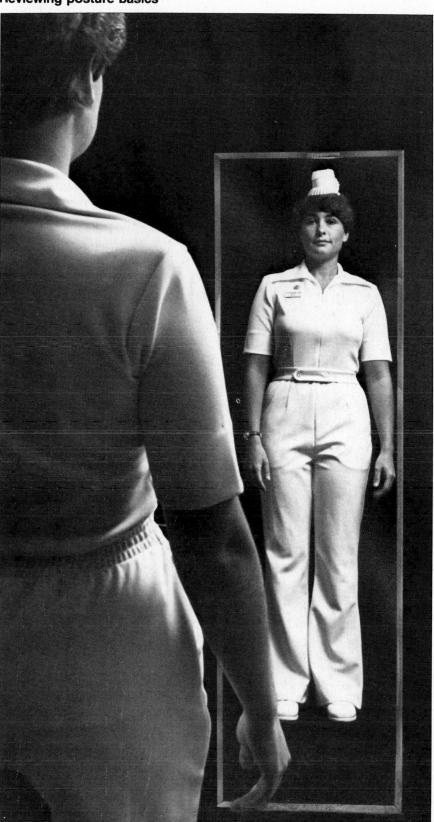

1 *How often do you say to yourself, "I really should improve my posture"?*

As you know, maintaining correct posture helps you look more confident, stand longer hours without back strain, and set a good example for your patients. Follow these steps to refresh your memory on posture basics:

First, stand in front of a full-length mirror. Keep your head erect, shoulders back, spine straight, and feet slightly apart. Pull in your abdomen, and slightly flex your knees. Move one foot in front of the other. Your muscles should feel relaxed.

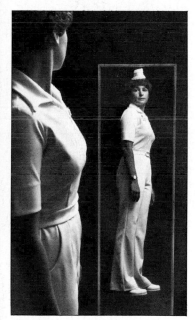

2 Now, turn to one side, and observe your body. Note your spinal curve: It should be slightly concave at the cervical and lumbar areas; and slightly convex at the dorsal and sacral areas. Make sure your shoulders are at an even height.

This position will enhance your well-being in two ways: by improving your circulation, and providing more room and support for your pelvic and abdominal organs.

Using basic body mechanics

Reviewing posture basics continued

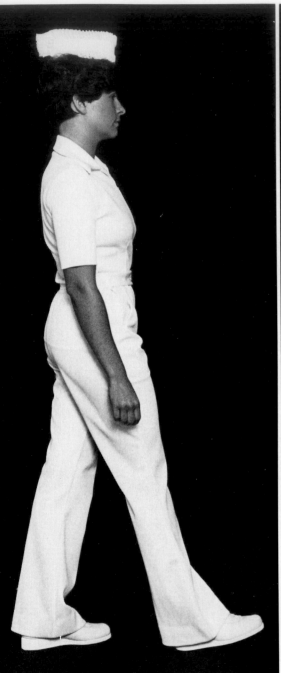
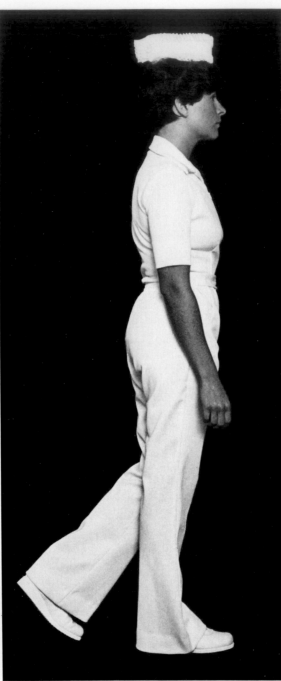
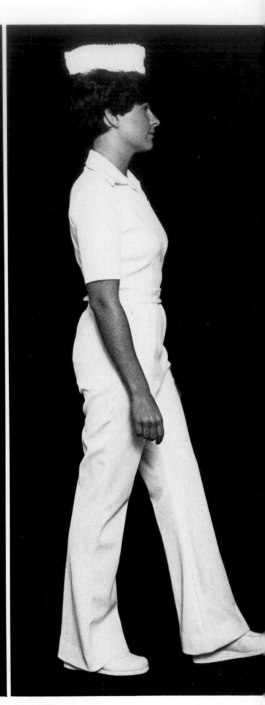

3 Next, using the posture basics you've just reviewed, try walking. Remember to keep your head erect, and your spine and pelvis straight.

As you step, let your heel, the ball of your foot, and your toes touch the floor in succession, as shown. Always keep one foot 6″ to 8″ (15 to 20 cm) ahead of the other.

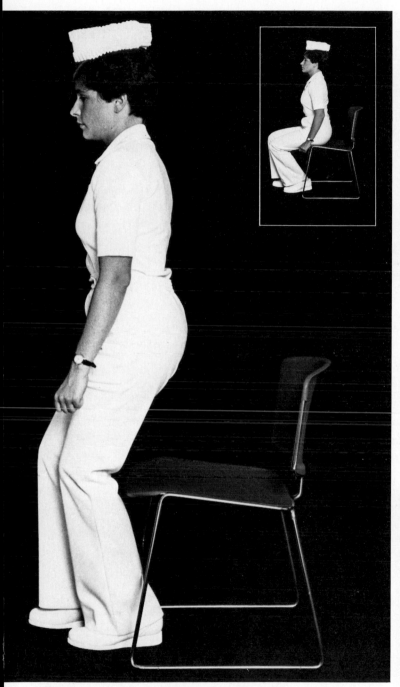

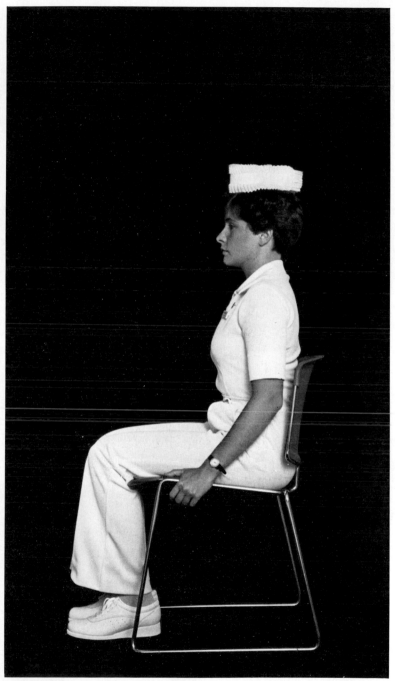

4 Now, you're ready to apply body mechanics to sitting. To do this, stand with your back to the front of the chair. Place one leg so it touches the chair and the other slightly forward. Keeping your upper body erect, bend at your hips.

[Inset] Then, using the calf muscles in the leg touching the chair, flex your knees, and lower your body. If the chair's low or deep, slide back in the chair. Reverse this procedure to get out of the chair.

5 Now that you're sitting in the chair, you'll want to position your body properly. To do this, hold your head and body erect. Keep your hips at a 90° angle to your trunk. Bend your knees, and place your feet flat on the floor, at a 90° angle to your legs. Make sure your weight's resting on your thighs and the widest part of your pelvis.

Using basic body mechanics

How to move an object, using proper body mechanics

Whenever you lift or move an object, first assess the object's size and weight. Carefully plan your movements; and make sure the path is clear. Then, follow these steps:

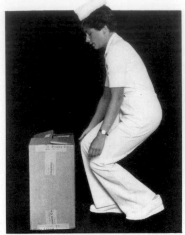

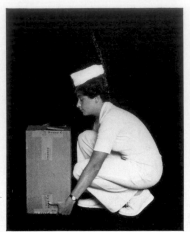

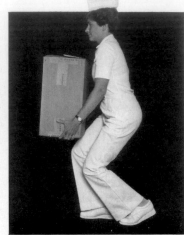

1 Want to lift a box from the floor? Stand facing the box. Widen your support base by positioning one foot slightly in front of the other. Keeping your back and upper body straight, lower your body by flexing your knees and hips, as shown here.

2 Next, move your center of gravity, which is located slightly below your waist, closer to the box. To do this, shift part of your weight to your advanced foot and part to the ball of your rear foot. Slip your hands underneath the box, as the nurse is doing in this photo.
Nursing tip: Always use your palms—not just your fingertips—to get a good grip on the box.

3 Keeping your upper body straight, use your leg and hip muscles to stand upright. Hold the box close to your body. *Remember:* The closer the box is to your center of gravity, the easier and safer it will be to lift.

How to use body mechanics to reach properly

Picture this situation: A hospital maintenance man has placed a large carton of heel and elbow protectors on a high shelf in your unit. Do you know how to use proper body mechanics to reach the carton? If you're unsure, follow these steps:

First, quickly assess the carton's size, approximate weight, and distance from you. If the carton's higher than your shoulder level, you'll need a stool or ladder to reach it. If you think the carton's too heavy for you to lift by yourself, ask a coworker to help.

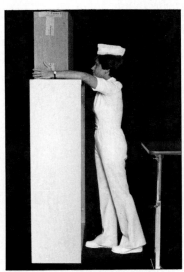

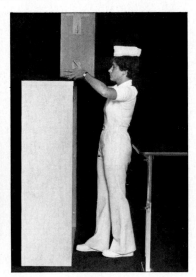

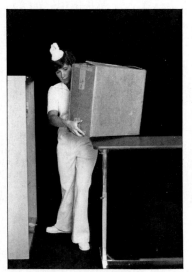

1 Now, stand close to the shelf, with one foot slightly in front of the other. Keeping your upper body straight and your knees flexed, place your hands on opposite sides of the carton.

2 Then, lift the carton, and bring it toward you.
Important: To prevent back strain caused by unexpected weight, never *slide* a carton off a shelf.

3 Next, using a smooth, coordinated movement, lower the carton to a waist-level table. As you do, keep the carton as close to your body as possible.

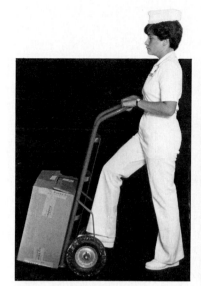

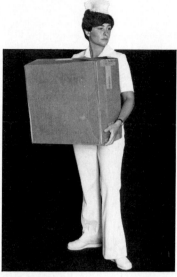

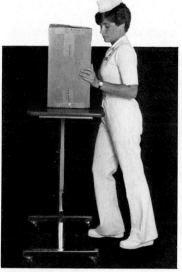

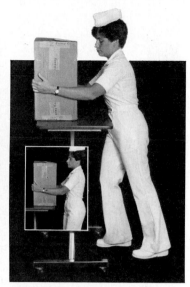

4 What if the box is too heavy or too large for you to lift by yourself. Ask a coworker for help. Or, use a hand truck, as shown in this photo.

5 Suppose, after lifting the box to waist level, you want to change direction; for example, to the left. Move your left foot, so your toes are pointing left. Follow with your right foot, turning your entire body.

Caution: Never change direction by twisting your back. Always move your *feet* first.

6 If the box is on a flat surface at waist level, you may be able to push or pull it. To push the box away from you properly, stand close to the table. Position one foot slightly in front of the other, keeping most of your weight on your *back* foot.

Place your palms on the side of the box closest to you. Shifting your weight to your advanced foot, lean toward the box, and *push* it with your body. Doing so adds body weight to your pushing force.

7 To pull the box toward you, stand facing it, with one foot in front of the other. Put most of your weight on your advanced foot. Place your hands on the back of the box. Then, shift your weight to your rear foot. Lean away from the box, and *pull* with your body (see inset). Doing so adds body weight to your pulling force.

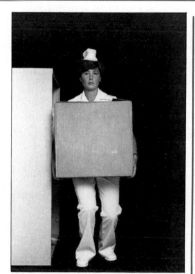

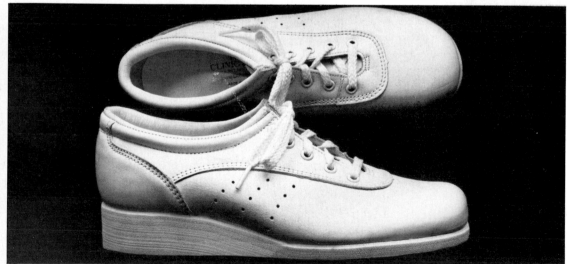

4 Suppose you want to move the carton from the table to the floor. Keeping your back straight, flex your hips and knees, and slowly lower the box to floor level.

Are your shoes safe and comfortable?
Maybe they're not, if they have open backs or wooden soles.

As you know, a good support base is essential to proper body mechanics. You'll need well-fitting, comfortable shoes— for example, Clinic®—to give you this base. Check your shoes, and make sure they have:
• nonslip flexible soles

• a snug fit (correct width and length)
• closed backs.

Remember: Well-fitting shoes will help prevent slips, stumbles, and ankle turns.

Turning and positioning

How much do you know about turning and positioning? Do you know how to set up a positioning schedule? Or how to support your patient's hips with trochanter rolls?

On the next few pages, we'll show you many of the positioning aids available and explain how to use them. In addition, we'll review some of the pressure relief aids available and describe how they work. We'll tell you how to set up a positioning schedule to meet your patient's needs and show you a sample.

We'll also explain:
• how to use a drawsheet to move a patient to the side of a bed
• how to logroll a patient with a spinal injury
• how to use the bridging technique effectively
• how to reposition a patient
• step-by-step procedures for placing a patient in a side-lying and a prone position, as well as how to support a patient in a supine position.

Read these pages carefully.

Detecting immobility hazards

Chances are, you're familiar with many of the hazards of immobility; for example, contractures, decubitus ulcers, and pneumonia. But, did you know that immobility affects every body system? Study this chart carefully.

System
INTEGUMENTARY (SKIN)

Complications
• Painful, reddened areas
• Decubitus ulcers

Nursing intervention
• Turn and position your patient regularly, according to his needs.
• Observe *all* skin surfaces, especially bony prominences, for pressure signs, such as blanched or reddened areas.
• Keep your patient's skin clean and dry.
• When necessary, use special equipment to minimize pressure on your patient's body; for example, an egg crate, air, or water mattress; flotation pads; and heel and elbow protectors. (For more information on pressure relief aids, see pages 20-21.)
• Gently massage *around* (never on) pressure areas to stimulate circulation.
• From a distance of 18″ (45.7 cm), apply a heat lamp 15 minutes daily, if ordered. *Caution:* Check the patient's skin frequently to prevent burns.
• Whenever possible, avoid irritating your patient's skin by using a drawsheet or sheepskin to move him.
• Make sure your patient is on a high-protein, low-calcium diet, with plenty of fluids.
• Explain all procedures to your patient, and make sure he understands their importance.

System
MUSCULAR

Complications
• Contractures
• Decreased muscle tone
• Muscle atrophy

Nursing intervention
• Turn and position your patient regularly, according to his needs.
• Make sure his body's well aligned, and that his joints and muscles are properly supported.
• Perform complete range of motion at least three times a day.
• Use supportive devices, as needed, such as footdrop stops, splints, trochanter rolls, and hand rolls. (For more information on positioning aids, see pages 22-25.)
• Whenever possible, reduce edema by elevating extremities.
• Hyperextend your patient's hips at least three times daily.
• Explain all procedures to your patient, and make sure he understands their importance.

System
CARDIOVASCULAR

Complications
• Decreased myocardial tone
• Venous stasis
• Thrombus formation
• Orthostatic hypotension

Nursing intervention
• Whenever possible, place your patient in high-Fowler's or a seated position. If he's in a seated position, place his feet flat on the floor or on a footstool, to alleviate pressure on the backs of his knees.
• When seating your patient upright in bed, raise the head of the bed gradually.
• When possible, use standing transfers to move your patient from one place to another.
• Apply antiembolism stockings (TEDs), as ordered.
• Make sure your patient has a high-protein, low-calcium diet, with plenty of fluids.
• Gradually increase your patient's activities.
• Instruct your patient to exhale slowly when moving in bed to prevent him from performing a Valsalva maneuver.
• Explain all procedures to your patient, and make sure he understands their importance.

System
SKELETAL

Complications
- Backaches
- Osteoporosis from disuse

Nursing intervention
- Turn and position your patient regularly, according to his needs.
- Make sure his body's well aligned and that his joints and muscles are properly supported.
- Perform complete range-of-motion exercises at least three times a day.
- Periodically, try to stand your patient upright, or use a tilt table.
- Make sure your patient has a high-protein, low-calcium diet, with plenty of fluids.
- Check his urine for sediment, which may indicate early formation of renal calculi. If you note any sediment, send a urine specimen to the lab for analysis. Document the results, and notify the doctor, if necessary.
- Explain all procedures to your patient, and make sure he understands their importance.

System
RESPIRATORY

Complications
- Pooling of respiratory secretions
- Respiratory infections
- Hypostatic pneumonia
- Atelectasis
- Respiratory acidosis
- Pulmonary emboli

Nursing intervention
- Turn and position your patient regularly, according to his needs.
- Make sure your patient's body is well aligned and that his joints and muscles are properly supported.
- Encourage your patient to cough and deep breathe, to fully expand his lungs and clear secretions.
- Observe and assess your patient's respiratory patterns and breath sounds.
- Be prepared to administer IPPB treatments, as ordered.
- Encourage the use of incentive spirometry and blow bottles, as needed.
- Perform chest physiotherapy frequently.
- Percuss and vibrate your patient's chest to loosen secretions, as needed.
- Explain all procedures to your patient, and make sure he understands their importance.

System
GENITOURINARY

Complications
- Urinary retention
- Renal calculi
- Urinary tract infections

Nursing intervention
- When your patient needs to void, place her in a seated position to allow good urine drainage. If your patient's a male, have him stand, if he's able. Also, provide privacy.
- Observe your patient's pubic symphysis for bladder distention. If you suspect distention, palpate the area to confirm your findings.
- Minimize formation of new calculi by acidifying your patient's urine. Make sure he gets adequate amounts of vitamin C. Encourage him to drink orange or cranberry juice, or administer urine acidifiers, as ordered.
- Don't give your patient foods that leave an alkaline ash residue, such as tomato or grapefruit juice.
- Check his urine for sediment, which may indicate possible developing renal calculi. If you note any sediment, send a specimen to the lab for analysis. Document the results, and notify the doctor, if necessary.
- Explain all procedures to your patient, and make sure he understands their importance.

System
GASTROINTESTINAL

Complications
- Anorexia
- Constipation

Nursing intervention
- Make sure your patient has a balanced diet, with many of his food preferences and plenty of bulk. Arrange for your patient to have several small meals throughout the day instead of three large ones.
- Provide your patient with 1,000 to 2,000 ml of fluid daily, unless contraindicated.
- Be ready to administer stool softeners and laxatives, as needed.
- Check your patient's bowel movement history. If he's constipated, make sure his medication isn't causing the problem.
- Provide privacy for your patient when he's defecating.
- When possible, place your patient in a sitting position in a bathroom or commode chair.
- Gradually increase your patient's activities.
- Explain all procedures to your patient, and make sure he understands their importance.

System
NEUROLOGIC

Complications
- Dependency
- Disorientation
- Decreased motivation
- Insomnia

Nursing intervention
- Gradually increase your patient's physical activities. Encourage him to co-manage his care and to do as much for himself as possible.
- Hold frequent conversations with your patient to orient him. Keep him involved and informed on all aspects of his care and therapy.
- Provide your patient with intellectual stimulation. For example, suggest he receive visitors; read newspapers, books, and magazines; or work crossword puzzles.
- Avoid letting your patient take too many daytime naps.

Turning and positioning

Nurses' guide to common pressure relief aids

The best way to keep decubitus ulcers from developing is to minimize pressure on your patient's bony prominences and anticipate problems before they happen.

For example, if your patient's elderly, will be confined to bed for a long time, or shows signs of skin breakdown, consider using one of the pressure relief aids shown in this chart. If your hospital doesn't have one of these aids and you feel your patient could benefit from it, recommend the hospital consider ordering one.

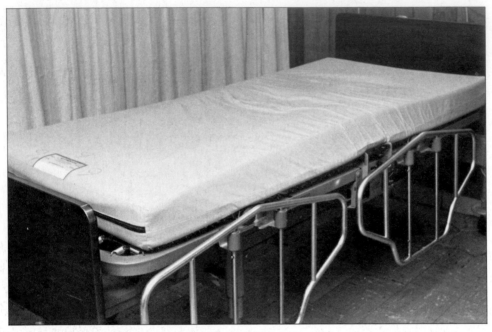

WATER MATTRESS

Function
• Reduces pressure by providing a water cushion between patient's body and bed frame

Nursing considerations
• Follow manufacturer's directions when filling mattress.
• Clean mattress with antiseptic solution before using it for another patient.

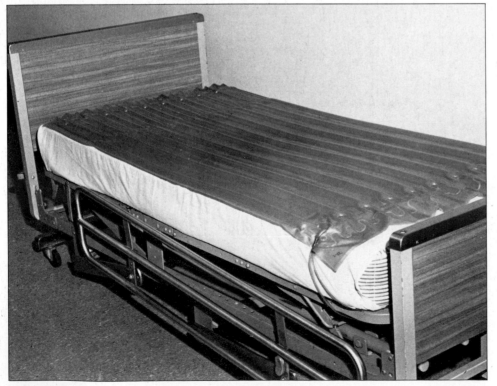

AIR MATTRESS

Functions
• Provides a comfortable air cushion between patient's body and bed mattress, thus minimizing the risk of pressure sores
• Some air mattresses are constructed so air circulates through them. With this type, the cushioning effect on the patient's body is enhanced, because mattress pressure is constantly being redistributed.

Nursing considerations
• Check to make sure the air mattress is inflated properly. If it is, you'll be able to indent the plastic approximately ½″ (1.3 cm) with your finger. Over- or underinflation reduces effectiveness.
• If the mattress is reusable, clean it with antiseptic solution, following your hospital's policy, before placing it underneath another patient.
• Avoid using sheepskin or a drawsheet with this mattress, because they reduce its effectiveness.
• If the mattress is disposable, discard it after one use.
• If you're using an alternating–air-current mattress, make sure all connections are secure and that the air pump plug is grounded.

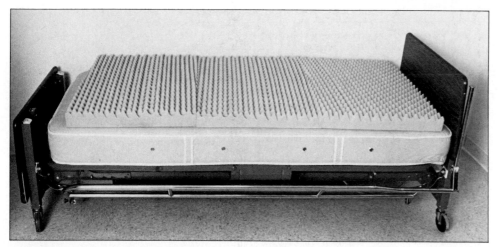

EGG CRATE MATTRESS (POSEY™ CONVOLUTED CUSHION)

Functions
- Reduces mattress pressure on patient's body
- Improves circulation of air on patient's skin

Nursing considerations
- If your patient's incontinent, cover mattress with the provided plastic sleeve.
- If mattress becomes wet or soiled, rinse it with water. Allow mattress to dry thoroughly before reusing it.
- Discard mattress after one use or send it home with the patient.

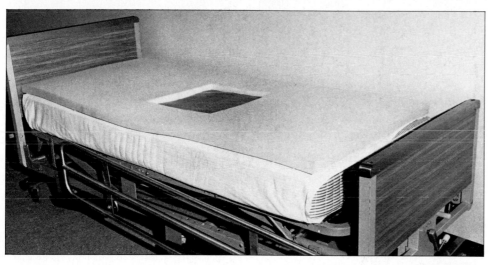

FLOTATION PAD MATTRESS

Function
- Reduces mattress pressure on patient's body and provides support by conforming to body contours

Nursing considerations
- Always cover flotation pad with the special cover provided or with a pillowcase.
- Never use a sheepskin with a flotation pad, because it will reduce the pad's effectiveness.

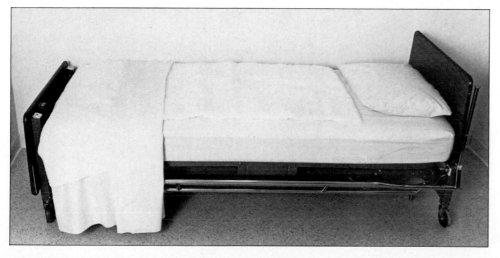

SHEEPSKIN (POSEY™ DECUBITUS PAD)

Function
- Provides soft padding to prevent pressure on the patient's bony prominences

Nursing considerations
- Position the sheepskin under your patient's heels, back, or sacrum.
- Make sure it's laundered, as needed.
- Impractical for sacral use if patient is incontinent.

Turning and positioning

Nurses' guide to positioning aids

To keep your patient's body aligned properly, you may need to use positioning aids. As you know, the number of aids you'll need to position your patient depends on his condition. Familiarize yourself with the more common ones by reading this chart carefully.

PILLOW (FEATHER, SHREDDED FOAM, OR FIBER-FILLED)

Possible applications
- Elevates extremity
- Supports patient on side
- Prevents pressure on skin

Nursing consideration
- In most cases, a pillow with a fabric cover (instead of plastic) works better, because it bends easier and is cooler.

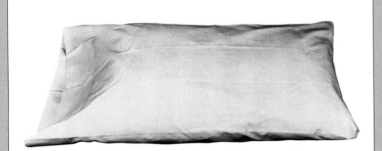

POSEY™ PALM GRIP (HAND ROLL)

Possible applications
- Helps prevent finger contractures
- Keeps hand and wrist in functional position

Nursing considerations
- Make sure hand roll's large enough to prevent finger flexion and to keep thumb in opposition.
- If hand roll slips out of place, secure it to the patient's hand with a gauze wrap. Fasten with tape.
- If a ready-made hand roll isn't available, improvise one by using a rolled washcloth.

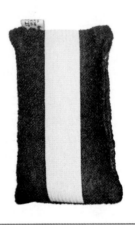
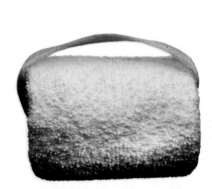

SPAN+AIDS® SCHAFER MODEL ABDUCTION PILLOW

Possible application
- Maintains hip abduction. Usually used after surgical repair of fractured hip.

Nursing considerations
- Make sure the pillow straps are padded. If they aren't, pad the straps with a small towel or a washcloth.
- Remove straps, and check skin surfaces for pressure spots every 4 hours, or more often if your patient's condition warrants it.
- Check tightness of the pillow strap by slipping your fingers between the strap and your patient's skin. Also, check his tibial and pedal pulses. Adjust strap, if necessary.
- When the pillow straps are in place, your patient may be turned on his side, or seated in a chair with his legs elevated and supported.

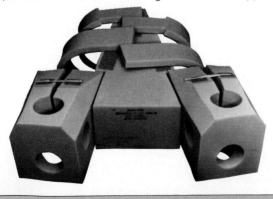

SPAN+AIDS® DELUXE CUT CRADLE BOOT

Possible applications
- Decreases mattress pressure on heel
- Helps prevent footdrop by keeping foot upright
- Helps control hip rotation

Nursing considerations
- Check your patient's skin color and temperature through the boot's opening.
- Remove boot at least once every 4 hours to check pressure areas.
- Patient may be positioned on side with boot in place.

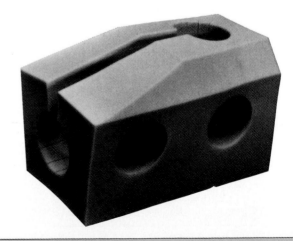

TROCHANTER ROLL

Possible application
• Controls hip rotation

Nursing considerations
• Make sure roll extends from patient's iliac crest to midthigh.
• If a ready-made trochanter roll isn't available, improvise one by using a rolled towel, bath blanket, sandbag, or pillow.

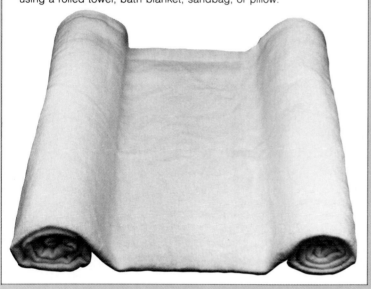

POSEY™ ADJUSTABLE FOOTBOARD

Possible applications
• Prevents footdrop by keeping feet in upright position
• Addition of antirotation blocks helps prevent hip rotation.

Nursing considerations
• If the footboard isn't padded, pad it with a towel or bath blanket.
• Apply heel protectors.
• Position your patient's heels over the mattress edge.
• Place your patient in a supine position for best results.
• If your patient continually slides down in bed, a footboard may be ineffective.

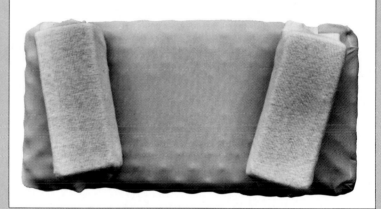

SPAN+AIDS® PRONE PILLOW

Possible application
• Supports prone patient's head and shoulders without hyperextending his neck

Nursing considerations
• Reassure your patient that the pillow will not suffocate him.
• Initially, use the pillow for only a short time, and stay with your patient until he becomes comfortable with it.

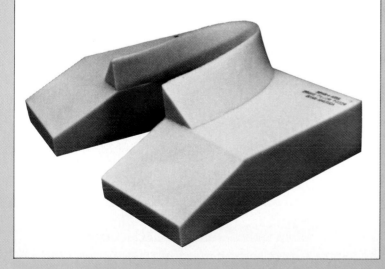

SPAN+AIDS® FOOTDROP STOP

Possible applications
• Maintains foot in functional position
• Helps prevent mattress pressure on patient's heel by elevating it
• Helps prevent foot rotation

Nursing considerations
• Patient may be placed in supine, side-lying, or prone position.
• Remove footdrop stop at least once every 4 hours to check for pressure areas.

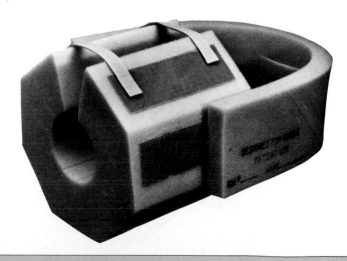

Turning and positioning

Nurses' guide to positioning aids continued

POSEY™ FINGER CONTRACTURE CUSHION

Possible applications
- Keeps fingers abducted
- Helps prevent finger contractures
- Gripping motions help increase hand strength.

Nursing considerations
- Remove at least every 4 hours to check for pressure areas.
- Have cushion laundered, as needed.

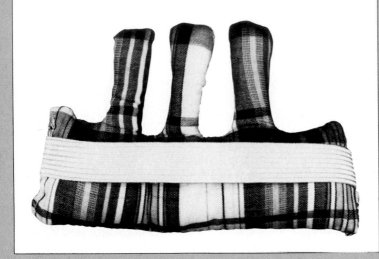

POSEY™ TURN AND HOLD SHEET

Possible applications
- May be used to turn patient from side to side
- May be secured to side rail to support patient in side-lying position

Nursing considerations
- Position sheet from patient's midthorax to below his hips.
- Have sheet laundered, as needed.

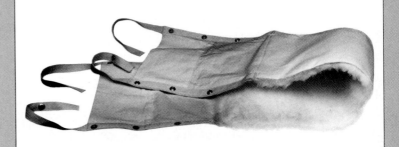

POSEY™ FOOT-GUARD

Possible applications
- Helps prevent footdrop
- Helps prevent foot rotation
- Keeps linens from pressing on foot
- Sheepskin lining helps decrease heel pressure.
- If necessary, plastic T-bar may be added for stabilization.

Nursing considerations
- Remove at least once every 4 hours to check for pressure areas.
- If your patient's positioned on his side, make sure the plastic heel's not in contact with his upper part of his leg.

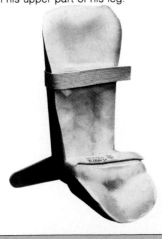

POSEY™ HEEL PROTECTOR

Possible applications
- Reduces mattress pressure on heels
- Helps reduce heel friction when patient's moved in bed

Nursing considerations
- Remove at least once every 4 hours to check pressure areas.
- Have the protectors laundered, as needed.

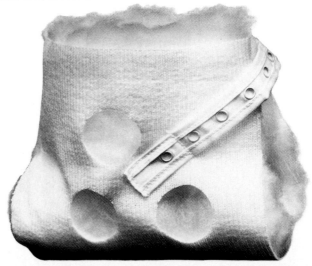

BED CRADLE

Possible application
- Helps keep feet free of linens

Nursing consideration
- Position directly over patient's upright toes.

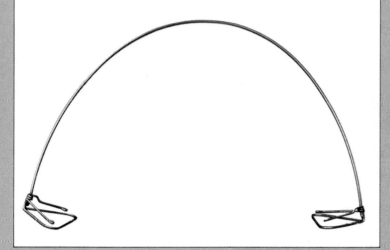

FRED SAMMON'S ARM SPLINT

Possible applications
- Keeps arm in functional position
- Helps prevent contractures

Nursing considerations
- Be sure to pad the inside of the splint.
- Remove at least once every 4 hours to check for pressure areas.
- Make sure splint doesn't press against other body parts.

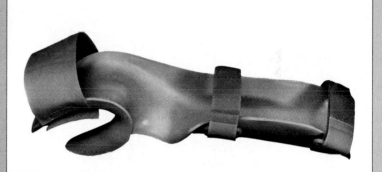

POSEY™ ELBOW PROTECTOR

Possible applications
- Reduces mattress pressure on elbows
- Helps reduce elbow friction when patient's moved in bed

Nursing considerations
- Remove at least once every 4 hours to check pressure areas.
- Have the protectors laundered, as needed.

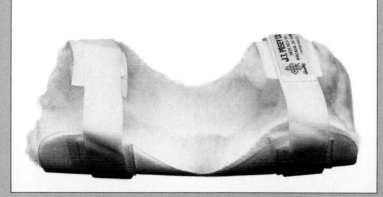

SCIMEDICS BELOW KNEE ORTHOSIS (leg splint)

Possible applications
- Keeps leg in functional position
- Helps prevent contractures

Nursing considerations
- Be sure to pad the inside of the splint.
- Remove at least once every 4 hours to check for pressure areas.
- Make sure splint doesn't press against other body parts.

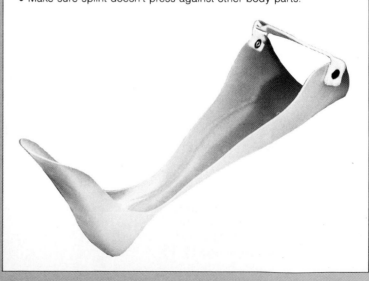

Turning and positioning

How to move your patient up in bed

1 *Picture this: You're ready to turn 31-year-old Carol Howard from a supine to a side-lying position. But, when you enter her room, you find she's slid down in bed. You'll have to move her up. Do you know how?*

First, raise the bed and lower the right side rail. Make sure the bed's in a flat position. Explain the procedure to Ms. Howard, and ask her to help you as much as possible.

Then, remove the pillow from under her head. Place the pillow at the head of the bed, as the nurse is doing here.

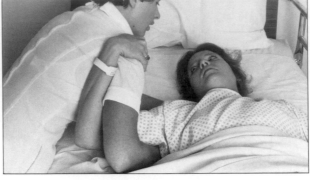

3 Now, hook your right arm under Ms. Howard's right axilla. Tell her to grasp your upper right arm and shoulder, as shown here.

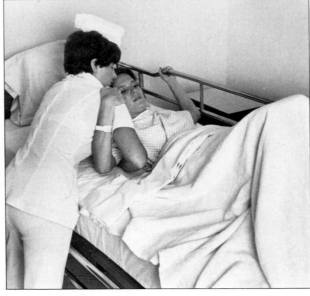

4 If possible, ask Ms. Howard to hold the left side rail with her left hand. Tell her to flex her knees and place her feet flat on the bed.

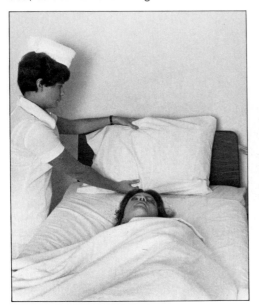

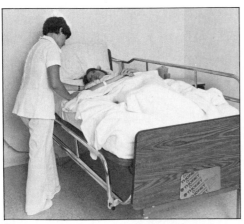

2 Position yourself on the right side of the bed, facing the headboard. Place one foot slightly in front of the other, and flex your knees. Remember to keep most of your weight on your back foot.

Bending at your waist, hips, and knees, lower yourself until you're close to Ms. Howard.

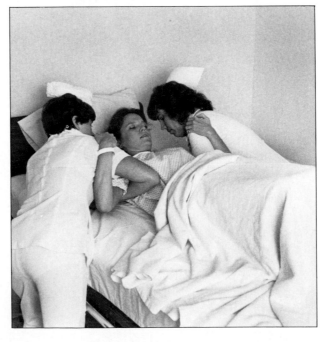

5 If your patient's heavy or very weak, ask a coworker to help you. Instruct your coworker to properly position herself on the left side of the bed. Then, tell her to hook her left arm under your patient's left axilla.

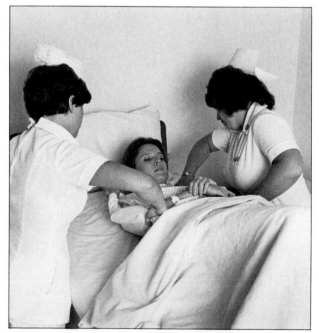

6 On a predetermined signal, instruct Ms. Howard to push down with her feet, raise her buttocks, and pull with her left arm.

As she does this, carefully slide Ms. Howard up. *Remember:* Encourage your patient to help as much as possible. However, if she can't, or if she has sacral skin breakdown, you may want to use the drawsheet method to move her up in bed.

7 To do this, make sure the drawsheet extends from her head to below her buttocks.

Ask a coworker for assistance, and tell her to position herself on the left side of the bed. Position yourself on the right side of the bed. Lower both side rails. Roll the long sides of the sheet close to your patient.

With one hand, firmly grasp the sheet near Ms. Howard's neck. With your other hand, grasp the sheet near her lower back. Instruct your coworker to do the same.

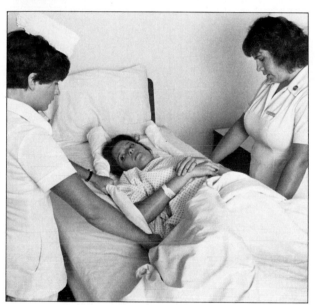

8 Flex your knees, and keep your back as straight as possible. Now, rock forward, shifting your weight from your back foot to your forward foot as you pull the drawsheet and Ms. Howard up.

Can your patient help you? On a predetermined signal, ask her to push with her feet and to lift her buttocks. At the same time, you and your coworker pull the drawsheet.

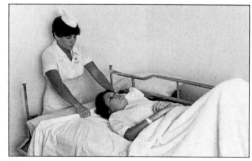

9 Suppose your hospital's short-staffed. You may have to move your patient up in bed *without assistance*. To do this, stand at the head of the bed, and detach the headboard (if possible). Check to make sure the drawsheet extends from your patient's shoulders to below her buttocks.

Important: Don't use this method unless your patient can bend her knees and push up with her feet.

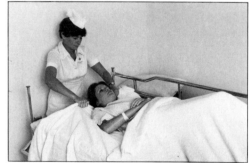

10 Grasp the sheet's edges near your patient's shoulders. Position one foot in front of the other. Rocking back on your feet, pull the sheet. Instruct your patient to bend her knees and to push up with her feet. This will prevent her heels from dragging on the bed.

■ *Nursing tip:* Changing the linens on your patient's bed? Loosen the bottom sheet around the entire bed, and use it to move your patient up in bed, as already explained.

Turning and positioning

Developing a positioning and skin care schedule

Wondering how to set up a positioning and skin care plan for your patient? You'll have to carefully assess your patient's condition, as well as his daily activities, including any scheduled therapies. Then, talk to your patient, and check his care plan.

Remember, a good positioning and skin care schedule will prevent complications and make your patient as comfortable as possible.

To the right, you'll find a sample positioning schedule and some helpful tips to help you develop a schedule tailored to your patient's individual needs. Here are the guidelines:

• Plan position changes and skin care around your patient's activities, and encourage him to participate as much as possible in developing the schedule. For example, does he want to be sitting up when he receives visitors? When does he usually have a bowel movement? When are his meals and medical treatments?

• Before implementing the schedule, ask the doctor to check it. You'll want to know whether any of the positions or positioning aids you've chosen may be contraindicated.

• *Important:* Use your common sense. Some patients may need to be turned more often than at the normal 2- to 3-hour intervals, and some may tolerate a position slightly longer. For example, if you note any blanched or reddened areas on your patient's skin, turn him immediately and adjust his schedule.

• Document the positioning schedule on your patient's care plan, and keep a copy at his bedside, for easy access.

• Be ready to revise the schedule at *any* time, as your patient's mental or physical condition improves (or deteriorates).

• Observe each position's effectiveness. Note whether joint motion is being decreased, maintained, or increased.

Remember, a good schedule always takes into consideration your patient's activities and how your patient feels. Develop your plan accordingly.

Sample positioning schedule

Patient's name: Bruce Johnson

Doctor: Charles Blackman, M.D.

Hospital identification number: 78910

Room: 232 Bed A

Time 9/8-9/9/80	Position	Notes
6 AM-7 AM	Right side-lying	Sleeping
7 AM-8 AM	Sitting in bed	Fed self breakfast
8 AM-10 AM	Supine	Complete bath given — ROM to all extremities
10 AM-11 AM	Left side-lying	Left unit to go to Physical Therapy Dept.
11 AM-1 PM	Sitting in chair	Fed self lunch
1 PM-2 PM	Prone	ROM to all extremities - tolerates prone position well M.O., RN
2 PM-4 PM	Right side-lying	Visiting with family
4 PM-6 PM	Sitting in wheelchair	Fed self dinner
6 PM-8 PM	Left side-lying	Visiting with friends
8 PM-9 PM	Prone	ROM to all extremities - evening care given
9 PM-11 PM	Right side-lying	Reading and watching TV - ROM to all extremities H.N., B.M.V
11 PM-3 AM	Supine	Sleeping
3 AM-6 AM	Left side-lying	Sleeping B.M.V, RN
M.O.- Mary Obenrader, RN HN - Helene Nawrocki, RN		B.M.V - Barbara McVan, RN

How to support a patient in a supine position

1 *Let's say you've placed Mary Quick, a 27-year-old telephone operator, flat on her back. Ms. Quick is a quadriplegic as the result of a car accident. You'll want to be sure her body's supported properly. Here's what to do:*

First, gather the following equipment: flat pillows; two footdrop guards, or a footboard with heel protectors; two trochanter rolls; and two hand rolls.

Then, make sure Ms. Quick's body is properly aligned with her arms straight at her sides. Check to be certain that her knees and toes point toward the ceiling.

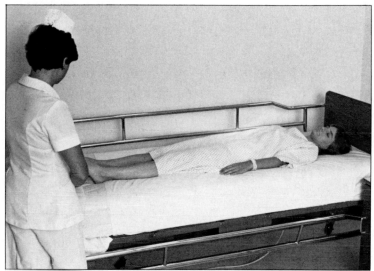

3 Suppose you're using a footboard. Position Ms. Quick's heels slightly over the mattress, in the space between the mattress and the footboard.

Then, place a small flat pillow or towel under her ankles.

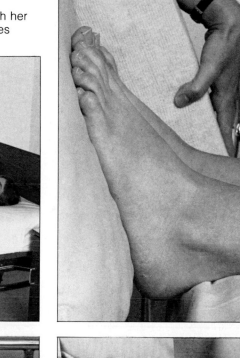

2 To prevent footdrop, use two footdrop guards or a footboard to properly support Ms. Quick's feet.

In this photostory, the nurse is using a Posey™ Foot-Guard. To apply it, place Ms. Quick's foot in the sheep-skin-lined plastic shell. Secure the shell with the attached Velcro straps. Then, attach the T-bar stabilizer to maintain her foot in the desired position. Position a small flat pillow or towel under each of her ankles.

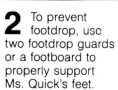

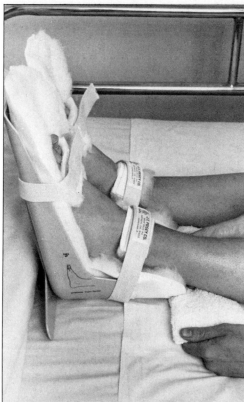

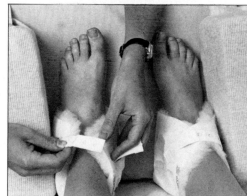

4 If insufficient space exists between the mattress and footboard, place heel protectors on both her feet.

5 Now, place a flat pillow under Ms. Quick's head. Avoid using an overstuffed pillow, as it may cause a flexion contracture of your patient's neck.

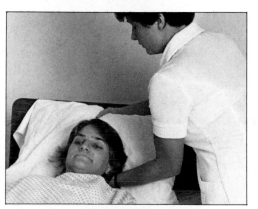

Turning and positioning

How to support a patient in a supine position continued

6 Because she's dependent, you'll also have to position her arms. Position a hand roll diagonally in each of her palms, with her thumb and fingers opposing each other, and abduct both arms in a palm-up position.

[Inset] Alternately, you may use a forearm and hand splint to keep Ms. Quick's hand and fingers aligned.

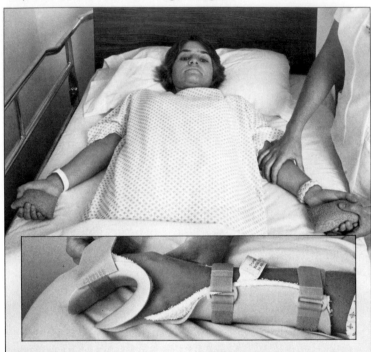

7 Or, abduct her right arm so it's at a 90° angle to her body, and position her left arm so it's fully extended at her side. Flex her right elbow so her forearm is pointing up at a 90° angle to her upper arm. Tuck a folded pillow under her right forearm, and place her hand in a palm-up position. Alternate the position of your patient's arms approximately every hour, depending on her condition.

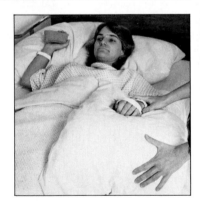

8 Another way to position arms is to place them at 90° angles to her body. Flex both elbows so each forearm's pointing down at a 90° angle to her upper arm. Put a folded pillow under each arm, and make sure each hand's in a palm-down position.

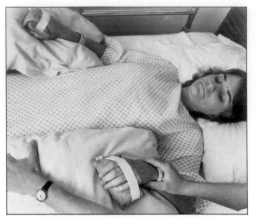

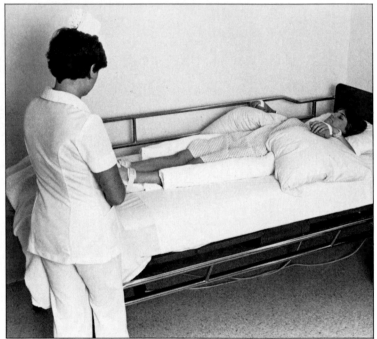

9 Next, tuck two trochanter rolls at the outer edges of her right and left hips to prevent external hip rotation.

Finally, cover Ms. Quick with a sheet or blanket and raise the side rail. Document how you changed Ms. Quick's position, as well as the date and time, in her care plan and positioning schedule.

The bridging technique: A way to reduce skin pressure

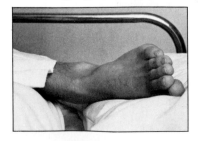

Anytime you want to reduce pressure on one of your patient's bony prominences, use the bridging technique. Here's an example:

Suppose your patient has a decubitus ulcer or reddened area on his ankle. Suspend the ankle between foam rubber cushions or pillows by position-

ing them above and below the ankle's bony prominences. As you can see, the bony prominences will then rest in the space between the two pillows (bridging). If necessary, use additional pillows or cushions to keep your patient's body in proper alignment.

Important: Never place a

pillow or cushion directly under a decubitus ulcer or reddened area.

As you know, when you use bridging, you'll still be able to turn your patient according to his positioning schedule. But remember, when you reposition him, you'll have to readjust the pillows or cushions.

How to place your patient in a side-lying position

1 *Do you know how to turn a dependent patient from a back-lying to a left side-lying position? This photostory will show you.*

Remember: If you want to turn your patient to a *right* side-lying position, follow the same steps, reversing the directions.

First, explain the procedure to your patient. Then, gather the following equipment: pillows, two hand rolls, a Span+Aids® Footdrop Stop, and a Span+Aids® Deluxe Cut Cradle Boot.

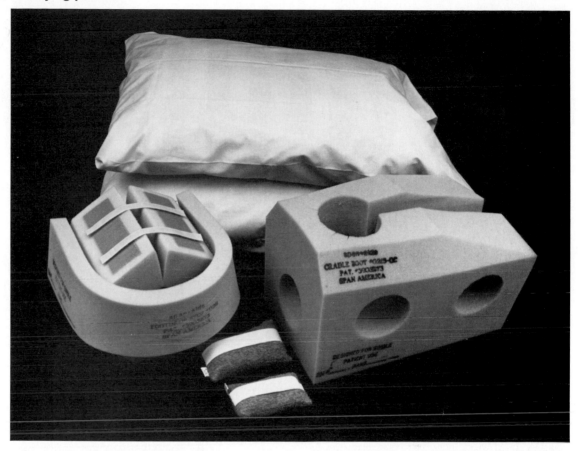

2 Now, lower the right side rail. Stand on the right side of the bed, facing your patient. Place one foot slightly in front of the other, and flex your knees.

Important: To ensure good body mechanics, always stand as close to the bed as possible.

If a drawsheet's positioned under your patient, use it to pull your patient toward the right side of the bed. To do this correctly, tightly roll the right side of the sheet close to your patient, as shown here.

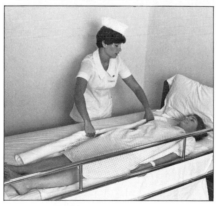

3 Then, firmly grasp the rolled end of the sheet with both hands. Gently pull the sheet and your patient toward you. As you do, rock back on your feet.

Finally, raise the right side rail.

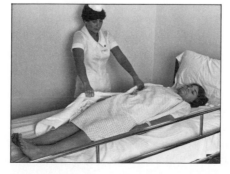

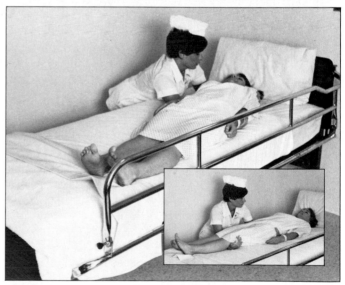

4 Suppose you don't have a drawsheet. Then, slide your hands (palms up) under your patient's shoulders. Pull her shoulders and upper body toward you, as the nurse is doing in this photo.

[Inset] Now, slide your hands (palms up) under your patient's hips. Pull her lower body and legs toward you. Finally, raise the right side rail.

Turning and positioning

How to place your patient in a side-lying position continued

5 Next, move to the left side of the bed, and lower the left side rail. Face your patient. Place one foot in front of the other, and flex your knees.

Bring your patient's right arm across her chest, as shown here, and make sure her left arm's abducted.

An important reminder: Flex your patient's right knee, and cross her right leg over her left before continuing the procedure.

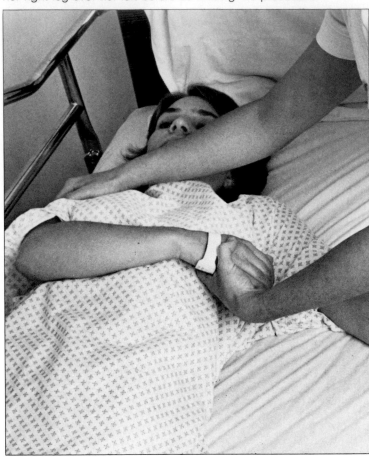

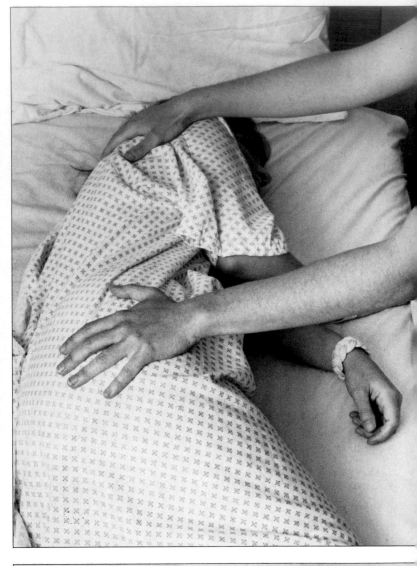

6 Place your right hand on your patient's right shoulder. Position your left hand on her right hip.

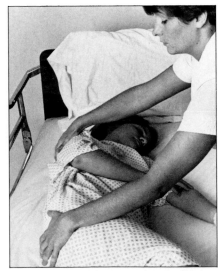

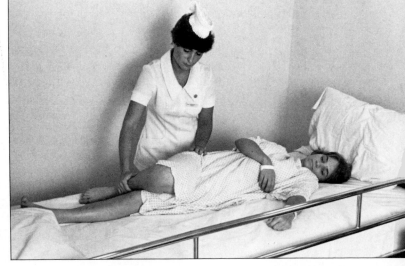

7 As you do this, rock backward, shifting your weight from your foot nearest the bed to your back foot.

Pulling with both hands simultaneously, roll your patient onto her left side.

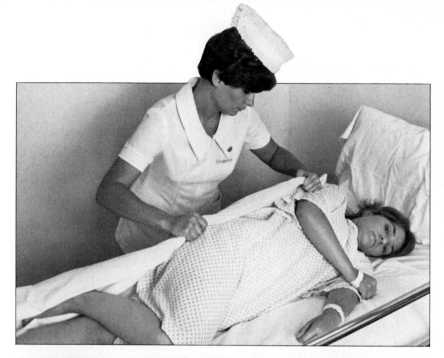

9 Now, tightly roll the right side of the sheet close to your patient. With your left hand, grasp the rolled end of the sheet close to your patient's chest. With your right hand, grasp the sheet near her hips, as shown here.

Slowly lift the drawsheet upward, rolling your patient onto her left side.

10 Tuck a pillow lengthwise behind your patient, from her shoulder to her coccyx. Make sure the pillow fits snugly against your patient's back.

Finally, raise the right side rail.

8 You may prefer to use the drawsheet method to move your patient from a back-lying to a side-lying position. To do this correctly, stand on the right side of the bed, as explained in step 2.

Then, bring your patient's right arm across her chest, and abduct her left arm. Flex your patient's right knee, and cross her right leg over her left.

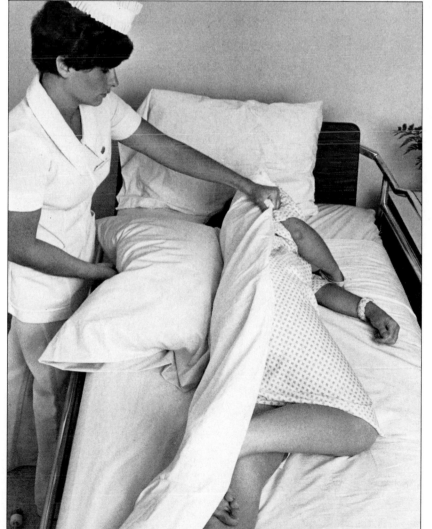

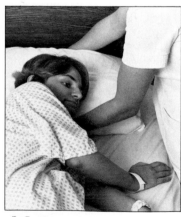

11 Now, place a flat pillow under your patient's head and neck, as shown in this photo.

Turning and positioning

How to place your patient in a side-lying position continued

12 Pull your patient's left shoulder toward you. Flex her left elbow at a 90° angle. Make sure her arm's abducted at approximately a 45° angle to the rest of her body, with her forearm resting against the pillow.

[Inset] Place a hand roll in her left hand.

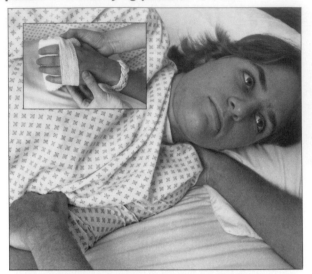

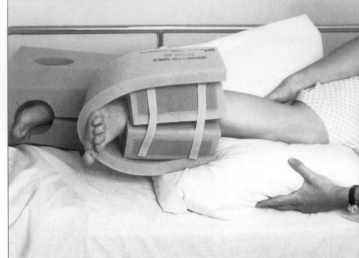

13 Now, place another pillow in front of your patient. Flexing your patient's right elbow, slightly abduct her right arm. Place a hand roll in her right hand, and rest her right arm on the pillow, as shown here.

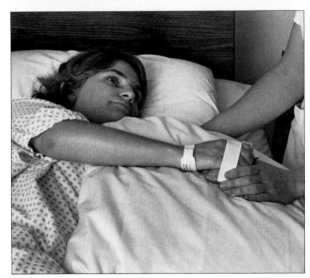

14 Carefully position your patient's left foot in a Span+Aids® Deluxe Cut Cradle Boot, as the nurse is doing here.

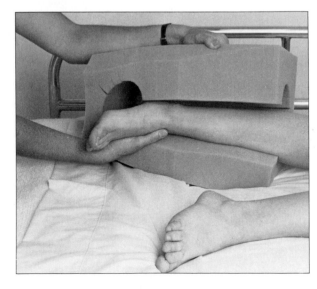

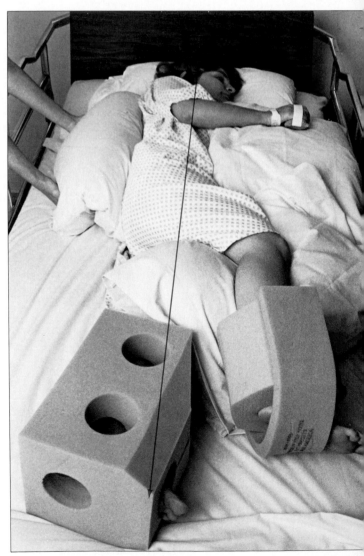

15 Position her right foot in a Span + Aids® Footdrop Stop.™ Then, place a folded pillow—or two pillows—under your patient's right leg and foot. If you're using a folded pillow, make sure the open edges face out.

16 Is your patient properly positioned? If she is, you'll be able to draw an imaginary line from the top of her head to the sole of her left foot.

Finally, document the position change, and the date and time on your patient's care plan and positioning schedule.

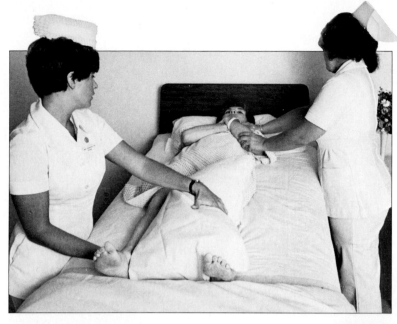

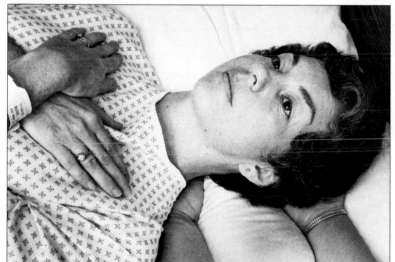

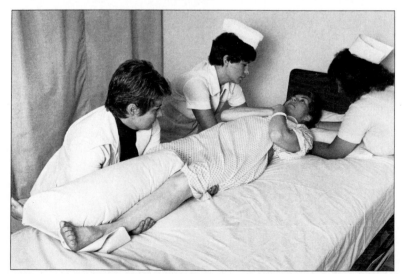

How to logroll a spinal-injured patient

1 *Are you caring for a patient with a spinal cord injury? If you are, sooner or later you'll have to move her from a supine position to a right side-lying position. To provide proper support and prevent further spinal injuries, use the logrolling technique. Depending on your patient's size, get the help of two or three coworkers. Then, follow these steps:*

Explain the procedure to your patient and reassure her. Raise the bed to your waist level, and lower the side rails. Make sure the bed is flat.

Position a pillow between your patient's legs. Cross her arms on her chest.

2 Now, ask coworker #1 to stand at the left side of the bed and to support your patient's head and neck, as shown here.

Important: Never permit a spinal-injured patient's neck to be twisted or hyperextended. This can cause further injuries.

3 Next, you and coworker #2 stand at the right side of the bed. Working together, extend your arms under your patient's shoulders, back, and buttocks. Then, on a predetermined signal, you and both your coworkers will simultaneously move your patient toward the right side of the bed. Or, use a drawsheet to do this, as explained on pages 32 and 33.

Turning and positioning

How to logroll a spinal-injured patient continued

4 Instruct coworker #2 to move to the left side of the bed. Tell her to position her right hand on your patient's right hip and her left hand on your patient's right knee. Place your left hand on your patient's right shoulder and your right hand on her right hip.

Coworker #1 should continue to carefully support your patient's head and neck.

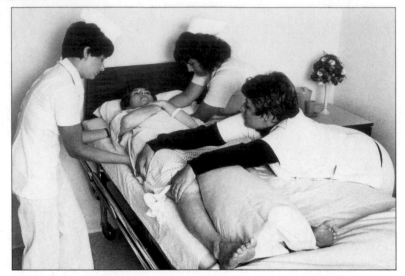

7 Or, complete this maneuver as follows: Stand on the other side of the bed, and turn your patient by reaching over her and grasping the drawsheet. Then, pull the drawsheet toward you, as coworker #1 continues to support your patient's head and neck.

5 On a predetermined signal, logroll your patient—as a unit—onto her left side. Keep her body perfectly aligned; never twist it.

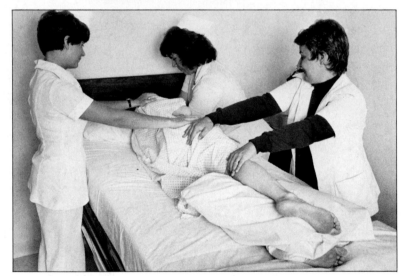

8 Finally, prop a pillow against your patient's back for support, and position her as explained on pages 31 to 34. Raise the side rails. Allow the pillow you've placed between her legs to remain there.

Document the position change, and the date and time on your patient's positioning schedule and care plan.

6 If you prefer, you can logroll your patient with a drawsheet. Instruct coworker #1 to stand on the left side of the bed and to support your patient's head and neck. Coworker #2 stands on the left side of the bed with her right hand on the patient's right shoulder and the other hand on her right thigh. Make sure the patient's body stays in alignment.

Stand facing the right side of the bed, and roll the drawsheet close to your patient. Grasp the drawsheet near your patient's shoulders and hips.

On a predetermined signal, lift the sheet up, rolling your patient onto her left side.

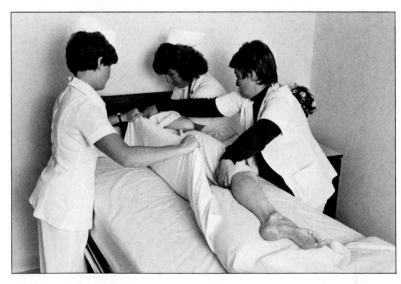

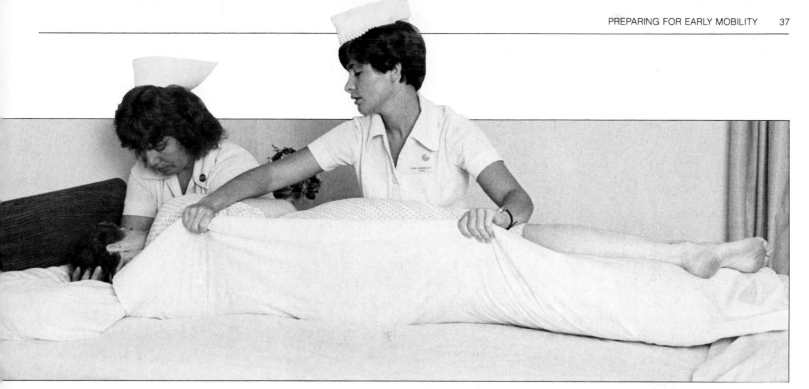

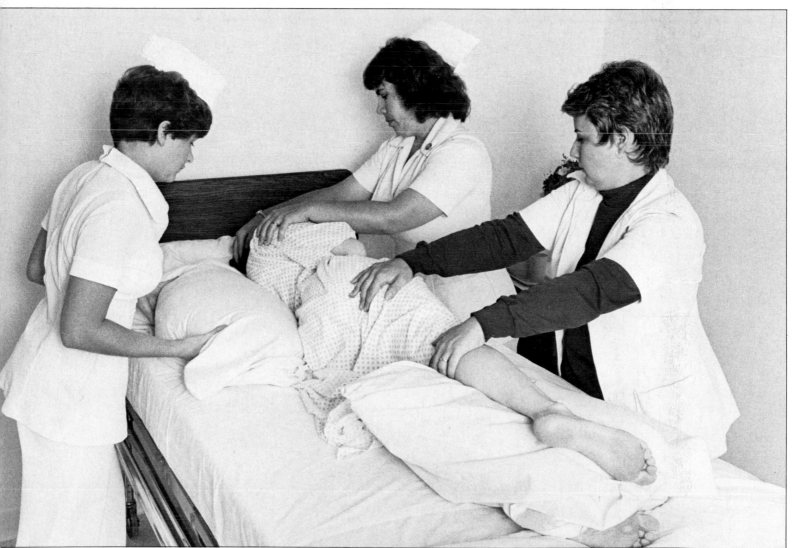

Turning and positioning

How to place your patient in a prone position

1 *Let's assume you're turning your patient from a left side-lying position to a prone position. Remember, the prone position may be contraindicated for some patients, such as those with respiratory distress, cardiac disorders, recent abdominal surgery, or severe hip contractures.*

Follow these steps to place your patient in a prone position: First, gather the following equipment: hand rolls, pillows, and shoulder rolls, or a prone pillow, if available.

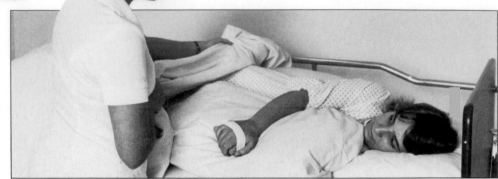

2 Then, raise your patient's bed to slightly below your waist level, and lower the right side rail. Carefully move your patient to the right side of the bed, as explained on page 31.

Next, remove any pillows or other supportive devices. Raise the right side rail.

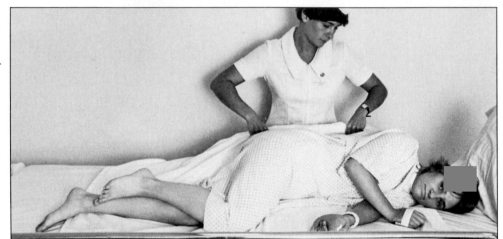

3 Now, move to the left side of the bed. Stand facing your patient, with one foot slightly in front of the other. Lower the left side rail.

Gently, straighten your patient's left arm. Position it (palm up) next to her left side. Tuck her left palm under her left thigh.

[Inset] Then, flex her right leg at the hip and the knee to make turning easier. Place your right hand on your patient's right shoulder. Position your left hand on her right hip.

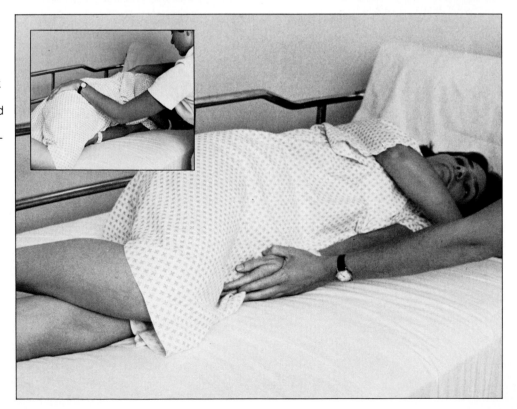

4 Flex your knees, and shift your weight to your back foot. As you do this, slowly roll your patient toward you, onto her abdomen.

Check to make sure her left arm's not caught under her body. Also, be sure she isn't face down on the pillow.

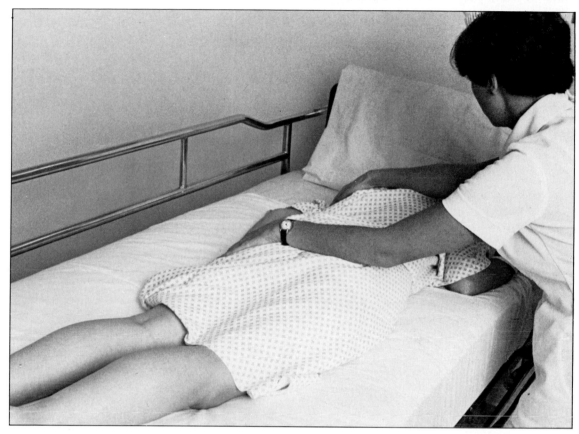

5 Is your patient positioned correctly? If she is, her body will be centered on the bed, with her feet hanging free between the bed and footboard.

Next, position a small flat pad under each of your patient's ankles, as the nurse is doing here.

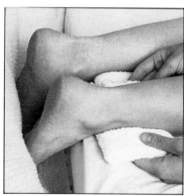

6 Now, abduct your patient's right arm, so it's at a 90° angle to her body. Flex her elbow up, positioning her forearm at a 90° angle to her upper arm, as shown here. Place a shoulder roll under her right shoulder.

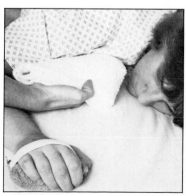

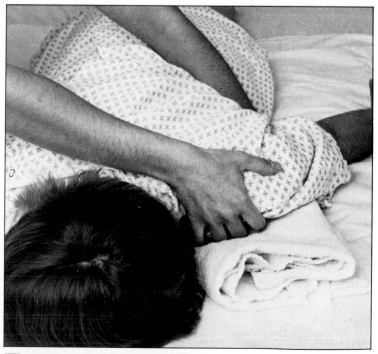

7 Abduct your patient's left arm. Then, turn your patient's head toward her right shoulder. Place a shoulder roll under her left shoulder, as the nurse is doing here.

Turning and positioning

How to place your patient in a prone position continued

8 When your patient's in this position, alternately place her left arm over her head; straighten and abduct her right arm. Turn her head to the right side.

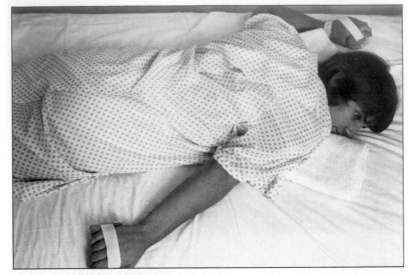

9 Or, abduct both arms, as shown here.
You can also position both arms on each side of her head. To do this, abduct her right arm so it's at a 90° angle to her body..Flex her right elbow up, positioning her forearm at a 90° angle to her upper arm. Follow the same procedure to position her left arm.

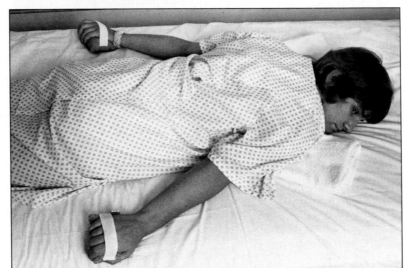

10 If you're using a prone pillow instead of regular pillows and shoulder rolls, position it under your patient's head and shoulders. The patient here is positioned on a Span+Aids® Prone Pillow. *Remember:* With a prone pillow, you won't need to position rolls under your patient's shoulders.
No matter which type of pillow you use, place hand rolls diagonally in both your patient's palms, as shown.
Finally, document the position change, and the date and time in your patient's care plan and positioning schedule.

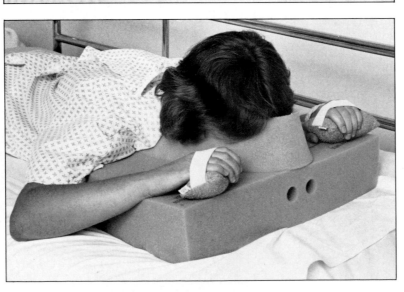

Moving a patient in traction

1 *You're working in the orthopedic unit and caring for 32-year-old Curt Roberts. Curt has his right leg in a Buck's extension device, with an overhead trapeze. When you enter his room to give him medication, you notice he's slid down in bed. Follow these steps to adjust his position:*
First, explain the procedure to Mr. Roberts, and ask him to help as much as possible. Make sure the bed is flat and a drawsheet's positioned under him. Then, ask two coworkers to assist you.

2 Now, position yourself on Mr. Roberts' right side, and lower the side rail. Tightly roll the drawsheet as close to him as possible.
Ask coworker #1 to stand on Mr. Roberts' left side and tightly roll the left side of the drawsheet as close as possible to him.

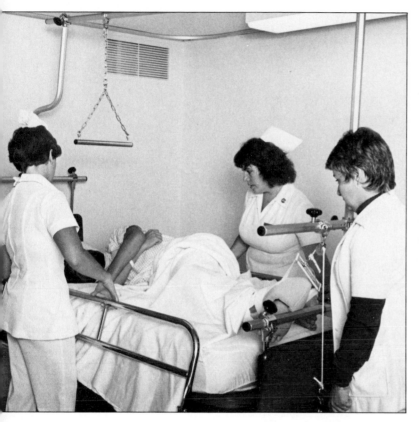

3 Instruct coworker #2 to stand at the foot of the bed and support Mr. Roberts' right leg, as shown here.

If Mr. Roberts is able, direct him to bend his left knee slightly and place his left foot flat on the bed. Then, ask him to grasp the overhead trapeze with both hands.

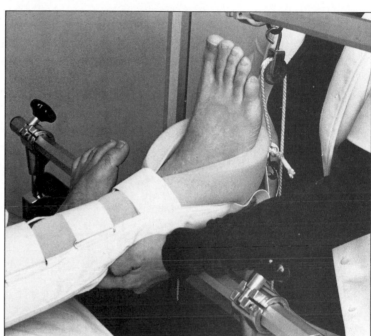

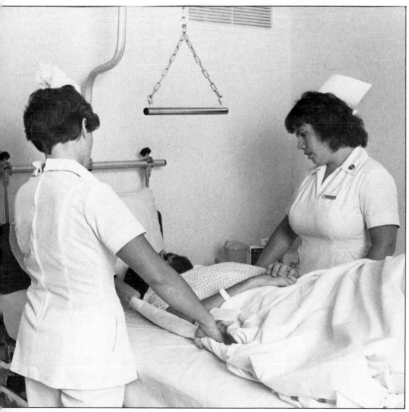

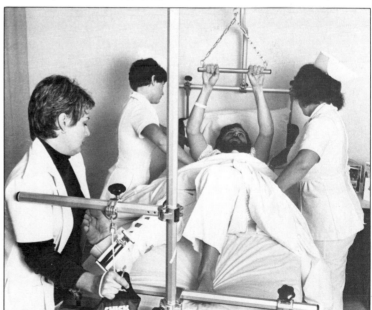

4 On a predetermined signal, tell him to push his left foot against the bed, as he helps pull himself up with the overhead trapeze. Then, simultaneously, you and coworker #1 gently slide Mr. Roberts toward the head of the bed. Coworker #2 will guide the weight at the foot of the bed.

Finally, document the position change in Mr. Roberts' care plan and positioning schedule.

Turning and positioning

Placing your patient in a leg-dangling position

1 *Has the doctor ordered your patient to dangle his legs twice daily? If so, you'll want to know how to place your patient in this position. Here's how:*

First, explain the procedure to your patient, and ask him to help as much as possible. Raise the bed to your waist level, and make sure it's flat.

Stand at the left side of the bed, with one foot slightly in front of the other. Make sure your patient's in a side-lying position.

Important: If your patient has hemiparesis, always roll him onto his uninvolved side.

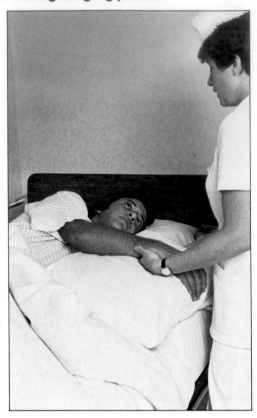

2 Instruct your patient to tuck his left arm under his side, flexing his elbow.

If necessary, give him additional support by placing your right arm under his shoulder and neck. Position your left arm under his thighs and behind his knees.

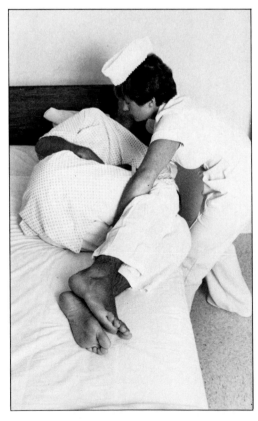

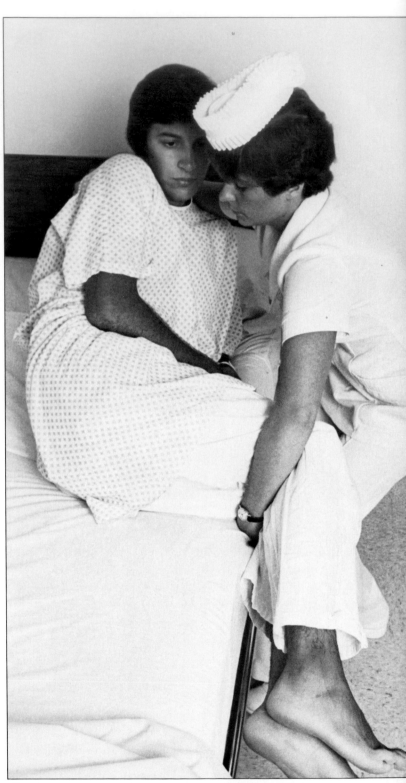

3 On a predetermined signal, pull your patient's legs off the bed, and slowly pull his shoulders up to a sitting position. Encourage him to help you as much as possible by pushing down on the bed with his left arm.

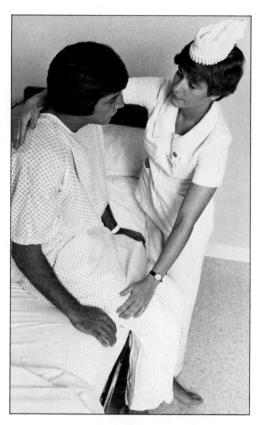

5 Continue to support his shoulders for a few moments after he's sitting upright. He may experience dizziness. Reassure him temporary dizziness is normal. If you suspect excessive dizziness—even if he doesn't complain about it—slowly lower him back to the bed. Then document the problem in his care plan and positioning schedule. However, if he has no dizziness, proceed as follows:

Lower the bed so your patient's feet rest flat on the floor. Or, rest his feet on a footstool.

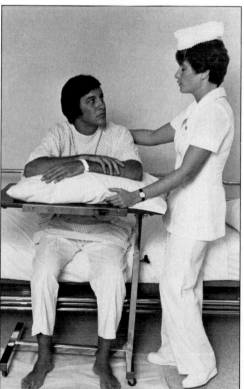

6 Instruct your patient to firmly grasp the edge of the bed, so he remains in an erect position. Continue to support him until you're certain he can support himself.
🕮 *Nursing tip:* Your patient may find it easier to support himself if he has something to lean on. Move an over-the-bed table in front of him, and place a pillow on it to make your patient more comfortable. Lock the table's wheels.

Finally, document the position change in your patient's care plan and positioning schedule.

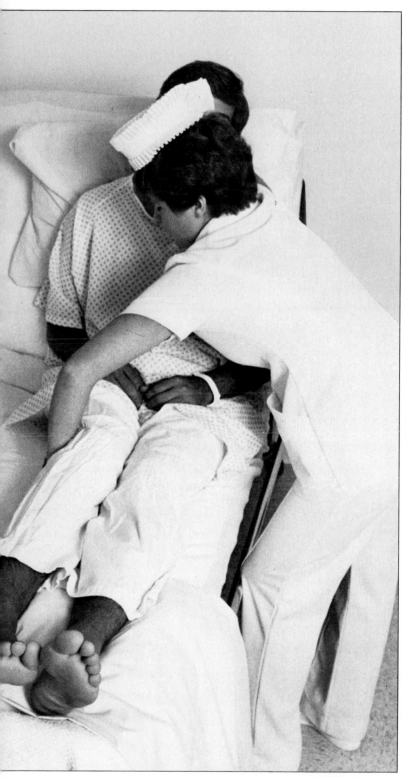

4 Here's another way to place your patient in this position. Slowly raise the head of the bed. Place your right arm around your patient's shoulders. As you lift your patient to a sitting position with your right arm, slide his legs off the bed with your left arm.

Turning and positioning

How to position your patient in a chair

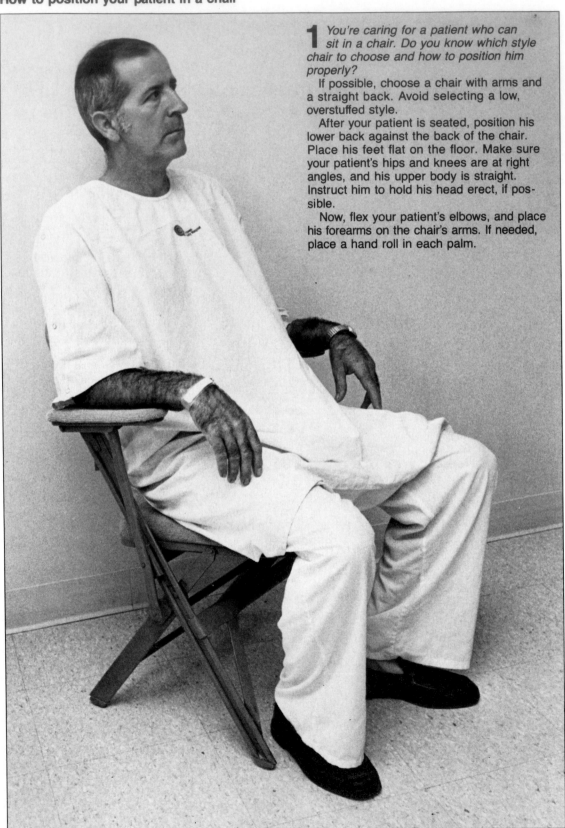

1 *You're caring for a patient who can sit in a chair. Do you know which style chair to choose and how to position him properly?*

If possible, choose a chair with arms and a straight back. Avoid selecting a low, overstuffed style.

After your patient is seated, position his lower back against the back of the chair. Place his feet flat on the floor. Make sure your patient's hips and knees are at right angles, and his upper body is straight. Instruct him to hold his head erect, if possible.

Now, flex your patient's elbows, and place his forearms on the chair's arms. If needed, place a hand roll in each palm.

2 If the chair doesn't have arms, or the arms are oddly shaped, you may have to place pillows or blankets under each of your patient's forearms for support.

Then, make sure his forearms are positioned at a 90° angle to his upper arms, as shown.

3 Suppose the seat of the chair is too deep. Place a pillow or cushion behind your patient's back.

What if the chair's too high. Get a footstool for your patient's feet. This will relieve pressure on the backs of his knees.

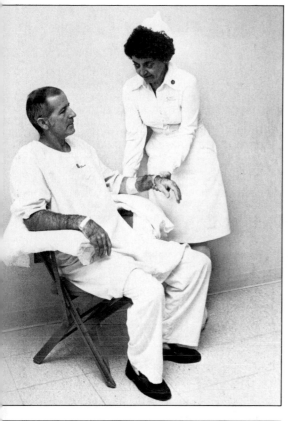

4 Is the chair too wide? Place cushions or pillows on both sides of your patient. Rest his arms on the cushions, as shown.
[Inset] If the chair's too low, place a cushion on the seat, as the nurse is doing here, and pad the chair's arms, if needed.

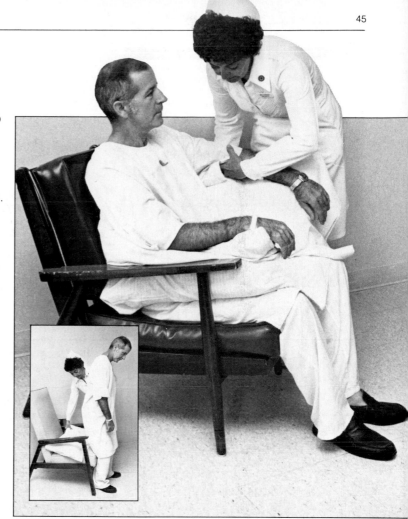

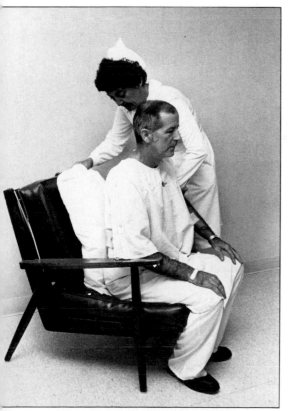

5 Finally, if your patient's having difficulty sitting upright, get a doctor's order to apply a vest or waist restraint. A waist restraint will prevent your patient from slipping out of the chair. The nurse in this photo is placing a Span+Aids® Safety Strap around the patient's waist.

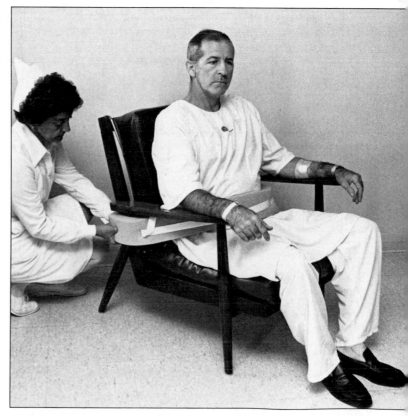

Reviewing exercises

Caring for a patient who has had a spinal cord injury or cerebrovascular accident (CVA)? In such a case, your patient may be partially or totally unable to move a joint or extremity. You'll have to perform range-of-motion exercises for him.

Which type of range-of-motion exercises does your patient need? Passive? Active assistive? Active? Active resistive? Do you know how these types differ? Can they be combined? When should you perform these exercises? How often?

If you're not sure of the answers, read the following pages. In them, you'll also learn:
• some precautions to take if your patient has a special problem; for example, amputation of a limb.
• how to teach your patient isometric exercises.

Reviewing basic terms
To help you better understand joint mobility and range-of-motion exercises, let's review some definitions of terms you'll be using.

Adduction: To move a joint or extremity *toward* the body's midline
Abduction: To move a joint or extremity *away* from the body's midline
Rotation, internal: To turn a joint or extremity on its axis *toward* the body's midline
Rotation, external: To turn a joint or extremity on its axis *away* from the body's midline
Flexion: To decrease the angle between two bones
Lateral flexion: To bend a joint to one side and decrease the angle between two bones
Palmar flexion: To bend the wrist forward
Plantar flexion: To bend the foot downward (also called hyperextension of the ankle)
Dorsiflexion of the wrist: To bend the wrist backward (also called hyperextension of the wrist)
Dorsiflexion of the ankle: To bend the foot up, toward the leg
Extension: To straighten a joint
Hyperextension: To move a joint past normal extension
Supination: To place the body, foot, or palm up
Pronation: To place the body, foot, or palm down
Opposition: To touch the thumb to each finger
Circumduction: To move a joint in circles
Inversion: To turn the foot in
Eversion: To turn the foot out
Radial deviation: To tilt an upright hand toward its thumb
Ulnar deviation: To tilt an upright hand toward its little finger

MINI-ASSESSMENT

Range of motion (ROM): How to choose your patient's exercise program
Have you ever wondered how range-of-motion exercises can aid mobility? When we talk about range-of-motion exercises, we're referring to a program that takes your patient's joints through their extent of movement and maintains joint functions. It also helps maintain muscle tone.

Has the doctor ordered any range-of-motion exercises for your patient? If so, you'll probably play an active part in planning your patient's program. Do you know which type of exercises your patient needs? First, consult with your patient's doctor and physical therapist. They may select your patient's ROM exercise program, depending on your hospital's policy. Then, ask yourself these questions:
• Is my patient unable to move his affected extremity? If so, he'll require *passive* range-of-motion exercises.
• Does my patient have only partial use of his affected joint or extremity? In this case, he'll require *active assistive* range-of-motion exercises. You'll guide him through these exercises, letting him assist you.
• What if my patient needs only to strengthen a weakened joint or extremity? Show him how to perform *active* range-of-motion exercises. In addition, show him how to perform any other exercises ordered by his doctor or physical therapist.
• Does my patient need more strength in specific joints or extremities; for example, to support his body while using a walker? Then, help him perform *active resistive* range-of-motion exercises.

Important: Before beginning any exercise program, be sure to check your patient's care plan, medical history, physical condition, and emotional status.

How to perform passive range-of-motion (ROM) exercises

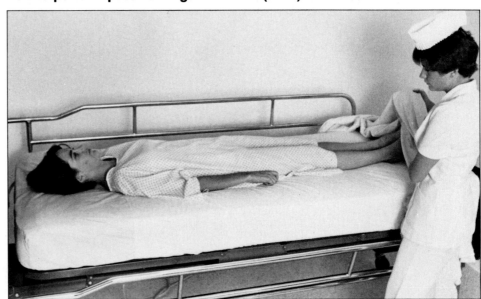

Getting ready to perform passive range-of-motion exercises for your patient? First, explain the selected procedure to your patient and reassure her.

Then, if possible, position your patient flat on her back, without a pillow. Place her hands at her sides and her feet together. Remove any sheets and blankets covering the joint or extremity you'll be exercising. But, keep the rest of your patient's body covered to keep her warm.

When you perform passive ROM exercises, always follow the right-to-left routine, shown in this PHOTOBOOK. Also, begin by exercising your patient's neck joints, and work down to her toes. Repeat each exercise at least three times.

Important: If your patient complains of pain during ROM exercises, stop immediately, and document this in your notes.

How to perform range-of-motion (ROM) exercises on your patient's neck

You'll need to guide your patient through five separate neck movements to correctly perform ROM exercises. Use the illustrated chart below for review. Then, read the following photostory for detailed instructions on how to perform each exercise.

An important reminder: If, at any time, your patient feels pain or you meet resistance when performing an exercise, stop immediately.

Caution: Never perform these range-of-motion exercises on a patient who has an abnormality of the basilar or the vertebral artery, cervical arthritis, or suspected neck injury.

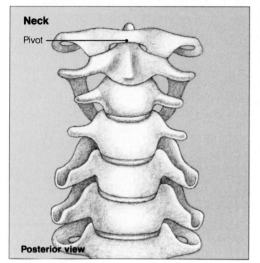

Neck

Pivot

Posterior view

Type of joint
• Pivot

Movement
• Rotation (normally, about 180°—90° each side)

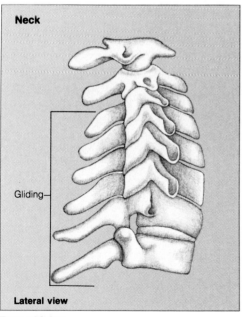

Neck

Gliding

Lateral view

Type of joint
• Gliding

Movement
• Lateral flexion (normally, about 30° each way)
• Flexion (normally, about 45°)
• Extension (normally, neck is straight in neutral position)
• Hyperextension (normally, about 25°)

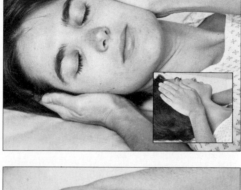

1 First, rotate your patient's neck joint. To do this correctly, position her flat on her back, without a pillow. Place your hands on both sides of her face. Turn your patient's head to her right until her ear touches the bed or as close to it as possible.

Then, turn her head to her left, using the same method (see inset). Repeat this exercise at least three times.

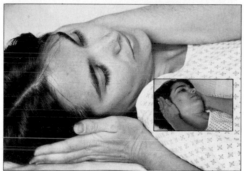

2 Next, we'll show you how to flex your patient's neck laterally. First, stabilize her shoulders, and place your hands over her ears. Flex her head and neck toward her right, as far as they can go comfortably.

[Inset] Then, flex her head and neck to her left, using the same method. Repeat this exercise at least three times.

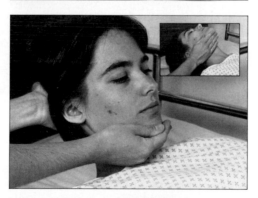

3 Here's how to flex and extend your patient's neck joints. Support the back of her head with your left hand. Move her head forward until her chin touches her chest.

[Inset] Then, move her head back until it touches the bed. Repeat this exercise at least three times.

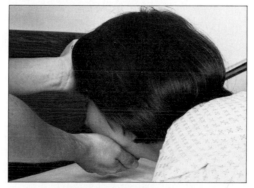

4 To hyperextend your patient's neck, place her in a prone position, or seat her on a chair. Support her jaw with your right hand and her forehead with your left hand, as shown here. Now, gently move her head back, and instruct her to look up. Continue to support her head as you allow it to return to the starting position. Repeat this exercise at least three times.

Reviewing exercises

How to perform range-of-motion (ROM) exercises on your patient's shoulders

You'll need to guide your patient through nine separate shoulder movements to correctly perform ROM exercises. Use the illustrated chart below for review. Then, read the following photostory for instructions on how to perform each shoulder exercise properly.

An important reminder: If, at any time, your patient feels pain or you meet resistance when performing an exercise, stop immediately.

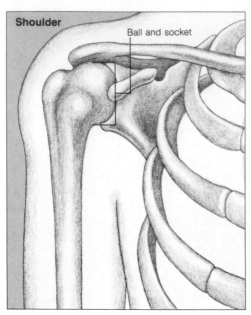

Shoulder

Ball and socket

Type of joint
• Ball and socket

Movement
• Adduction (normally, shoulder is straight in neutral position)
• Cross adduction (normally, about 45°)
• Abduction (normally, about 180°)
• Internal rotation (normally about 90°)
• External rotation (normally, about 90°)
• Flexion (normally, about 180°)
• Extension (normally, shoulder is straight in neutral position)
• Hyperextension (normally, about 65°)
• Circumduction (normally, about 360°)

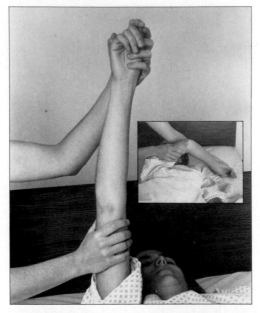

1 First, adduct your patient's shoulders. To do this properly, place her flat on her back. Then, put your right hand slightly above her right elbow. With your left hand, firmly grasp her right hand.

Now, raise your patient's right arm so it's at a 90° angle to her body.

[Inset] Slowly move her arm to the left (across her chest) until it touches the bed (cross adduction).

Then, bring her arm back to the starting position, using the same method. Repeat this exercise at least three times.

Follow the same procedure on her left shoulder.

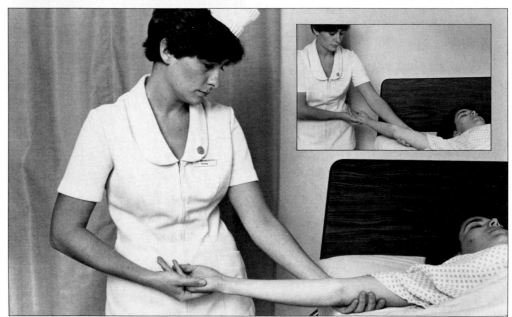

2 Here's an abduction exercise for your patient's shoulders. Begin by placing her right arm at her side, with her elbow straight and her palm up. Then, move her arm laterally, as shown in this photo.

[Inset] Continue moving her arm upward, keeping her elbow straight.

Suppose the headboard prevents you from raising your patient's arm with her elbow straight. In this case, bend her arm slightly at the elbow and continue. Or, elevate the head of the bed (if not contraindicated), and start the exercise again.

When your patient's arm touches the side of her head—or as close to it as possible—lower her arm to her side. Repeat this exercise at least three times.

Now, following the same procedure, perform this exercise on her left shoulder.

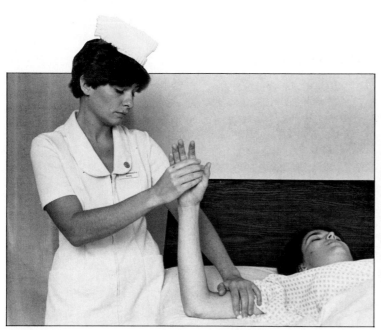

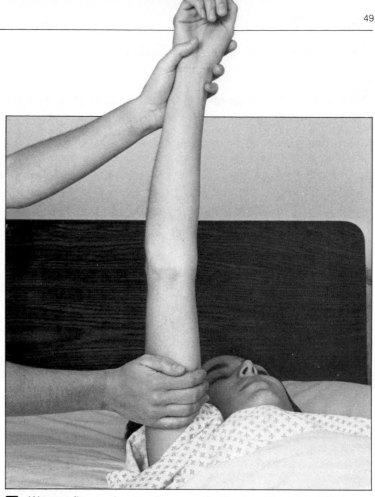

3 To rotate your patient's shoulder internally and externally, place your patient flat on her back. Then, abduct her right arm to shoulder level. Keep her palm up.

Bend her elbow, positioning her forearm perpendicular to the bed and her palm toward her feet, as shown here.

4 Keeping her upper arm and elbow against the bed, lower her forearm until her palm touches the bed. Then, raise her forearm so it's perpendicular to the bed.

[Inset] Now, gently guide your patient's forearm in the opposite direction, as shown here. When it touches the bed—or as close to it as possible—return her arm to its original position. Repeat this exercise at least three times.

Then, perform this exercise on her left shoulder.

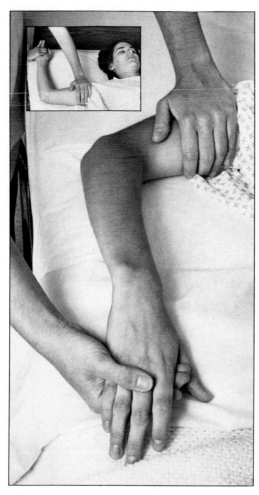

5 Want to flex and extend your patient's shoulder joints? Raise her right arm so it forms a 90° angle above the rest of her body. But, as you do, *be sure to keep her elbow straight.*

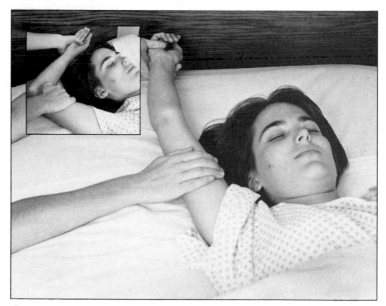

6 Gently move her arm back until the back of her hand touches the bed, or as close to it as possible. Remember, if the headboard prevents you from keeping your patient's elbow straight, bend her elbow to complete the flexion (see inset). Or, elevate the head of the bed, as before. Lower her arm to her side. Repeat this exercise at least three times.

Then, perform this exercise on her left shoulder.

Reviewing exercises

How to perform range-of-motion (ROM) exercises on your patient's shoulders continued

7 To hyperextend your patient's shoulder joints, place her in a prone position. Then, put your left hand on her left shoulder. Place your right hand under her left wrist.

Raise her right arm as far as possible. Then, return it to her side. Repeat this exercise at least three times.

Then, perform this exercise on her right shoulder.

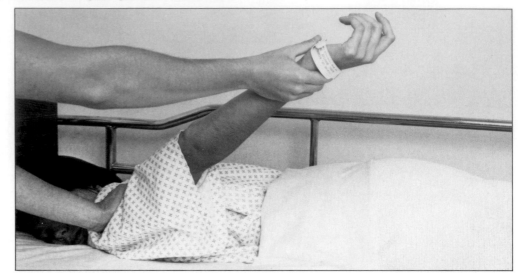

8 Taking your patient's shoulders through circumduction? If so, first make sure your patient can sit or stand alone. Then, position her so she can move her arms freely in all directions. Next, laterally raise your patient's right arm, with the palm forward, until it's perpendicular to the rest of her body, as shown here. Be sure to keep her elbow straight. Then, move her arm in a small circle.

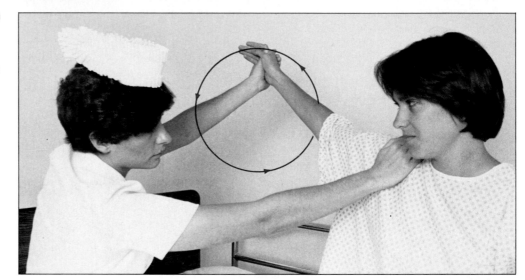

9 Now, move her arm in a larger circle, as shown here. As her shoulder mobility increases, increase the size of the circles. Repeat this exercise at least three times.

Then, perform this exercise on her left arm.

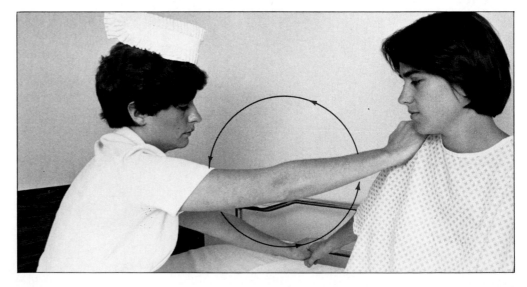

How to perform range-of-motion (ROM) exercises on your patient's elbows

You'll need to guide your patient through two separate elbow movements to correctly perform ROM exercises. Use the illustrated chart below for review. Then, read the following photostory thoroughly for detailed instructions on how to perform each exercise.

An important reminder: If, at any time, your patient feels pain or you meet resistance when performing an exercise, stop immediately.

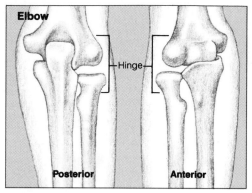

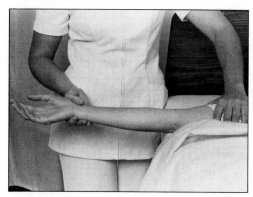

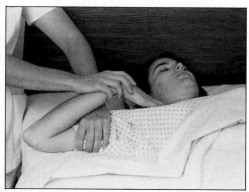

Type of joint
• Hinge

Movement
• Flexion (normally, about 145°)
• Extension (normally, elbow is straight in neutral position)

1 Here's how to flex and extend your patient's elbow. First, place her flat on her back. Extend her right arm to the side, with her palm up.

2 Bend your patient's right elbow, and guide her hand until it touches her right shoulder, or as close to it as possible. Then, straighten her elbow. Repeat this exercise at least three times.
   Then, follow the same procedure on her left elbow.

How to perform range-of-motion (ROM) exercises on your patient's forearms

You'll need to carefully guide your patient through two separate forearm movements to correctly perform ROM exercises. Use the illustrated chart below for review. Then, read the following photostory for detailed instructions on how to perform each exercise.

An important reminder: If, at any time, your patient feels pain or you meet resistance when performing an exercise, stop immediately.

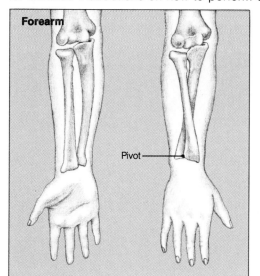

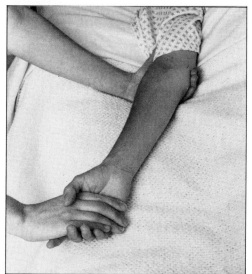

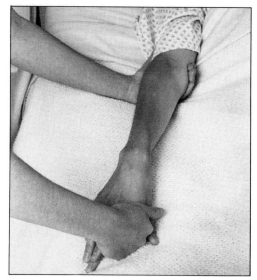

Type of joint
• Pivot

Movement
• Pronation (lower portions of radius and ulna rotate around each other; normally, distal ends rotate about 150°)
• Supination (normally, distal ends remain in neutral position)

1 Here's a pronation/supination exercise for your patient's forearms. First, place your patient flat on her back. Then, position her arms slightly away from her sides, with her palms up. Support her right elbow with your left hand, as the nurse is doing in this photo. Grasp her right hand with your right hand.

2 Turn her right palm down, rotating her hand and forearm, as shown here. Turn her palm up—then down—at least three times. Repeat this exercise on her left forearm.

Reviewing exercises

How to perform range-of-motion (ROM) exercises on your patient's wrists

You'll need to carefully guide your patient through five separate wrist movements to correctly perform ROM exercises. Use the illustrated chart below for review. Then, read the following photostory for detailed instructions on how to perform each exercise.

An important reminder: If, at any time, your patient feels pain or you meet resistance when performing an exercise, stop immediately.

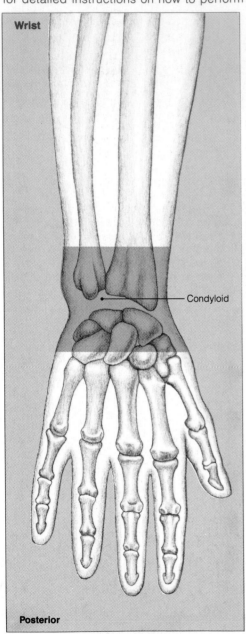

Wrist

— Condyloid

Posterior

Type of joint
• Condyloid

Movement
• Palmar flexion (also called flexion; normally, about 90°)
• Extension (normally, wrist is straight in neutral position)
• Dorsiflexion (also called hyperextension; normally, about 75°)
• Ulnar deviation (normally, about 45°)
• Radial deviation (normally, about 20°)

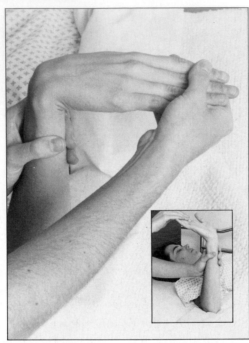

1 This photostory shows you palmar flexion, extension, dorsiflexion, and ulnar and radial deviation on your patient's wrists. First, position your patient flat on her back. Now, with your left hand, support her right arm just above her wrist. Use your right hand to grasp her right hand. Flex her hand forward, so her palm faces down, as shown here.

[Inset] Next, flex her hand back, so her palm faces up. Repeat this exercise at least three times.

Then, follow the same procedure on her left wrist.

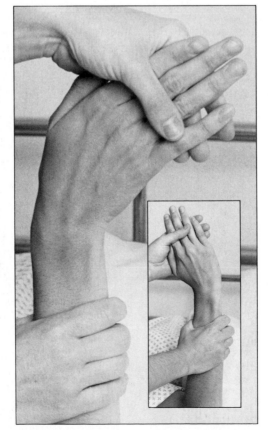

2 Now you're ready to perform the ulnar and the radial deviation exercises on your patient's wrists. To do this, support your patient's right arm just above her wrist. Move her hand to one side, as shown here.

[Inset] Then, move it to the other side. Repeat this exercise at least three times.

Then, follow the same procedure on her left wrist.

How to perform range-of-motion (ROM) exercises on your patient's hands and fingers

You'll need to guide your patient through 13 separate hand and finger movements to correctly perform ROM exercises. Use the chart below for review. Then, read the following photostory for detailed instructions on how to perform each exercise.

An important reminder: If, at any time, your patient feels pain or you meet resistance when performing an exercise, stop immediately.

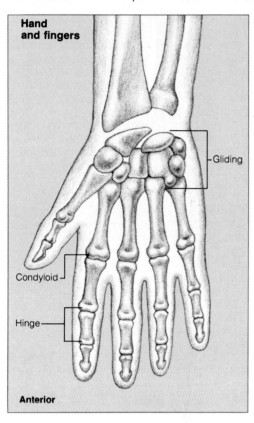

Hand and fingers

Gliding

Condyloid

Hinge

Anterior

Type of joint
• Gliding (palm only)

Movement
• Flexion (minimal)
• Extension (minimal)
• Adduction (minimal)
• Abduction (minimal)

Type of joint
• Condyloid (knuckle only)

Movement
• Flexion (normally, about 95°)
• Extension (normally, knuckle is straight in neutral position)
• Hyperextension (normally, about 12°)
• Limited adduction (normally, about 12°)
• Limited abduction (normally, about 12°)
• Circumduction (normally, about 360°, very small circular movement)

Type of joint
• Hinge (finger only)

Movement
• Flexion (normally, about 90°)
• Extension (normally, finger is straight in neutral position)

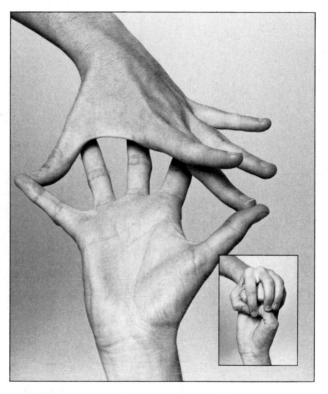

1 Here's how to flex and extend your patient's palm, knuckle, and finger joints. Support your patient's right wrist with your right hand. With your left hand, move her thumb away from her fingers. Then, push back evenly on her thumb and fingers.

[Inset] Now, place your left hand on top of your patient's hand, as shown here. Bend her fingers forward, curling them into a fist. Repeat these exercises at least three times.

Then, follow the same procedure on her left hand.

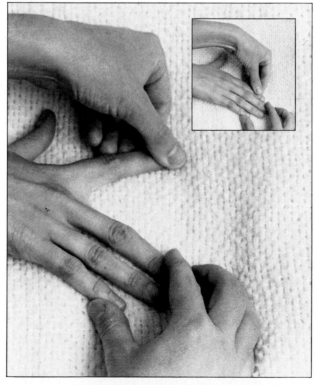

2 To perform adduction/abduction exercises for your patient's palm and knuckles, place her right hand on the bed, with her palm down. Support her fingers with your right hand. With your left hand, move each finger away from the adjacent finger, then back again (see inset). Repeat this exercise at least three times on each finger.

Then, follow the same procedure on her left hand.

Reviewing exercises

How to perform range-of-motion (ROM) exercises on your patient's thumbs

You'll need to guide your patient through 13 separate thumb movements to correctly perform ROM exercises. Use the chart below for review. Then, read the following photostory for detailed instructions on how to perform each exercise.

An important reminder: If, at any time, your patient feels pain or you meet resistance when performing an exercise, stop immediately.

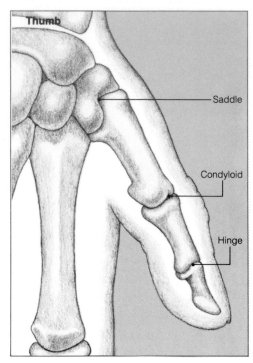

Type of joint
• Saddle (thumb and palm junction only)

Movement
• Extension (normally, about 90°)
• Flexion (normally, thumb is straight in neutral position)
• Hyperflexion (normally, about 45°)
• Opposition (normally, thumb can move toward little finger)
• Adduction (normally, thumb is straight in neutral position)
• Abduction (normally, about 90°)

Type of joint
• Condyloid (knuckle only)

Movement
• Flexion (normally, about 75°)
• Extension (normally, knuckle is straight in neutral position)
• Limited adduction (normally, knuckle is straight in neutral position)
• Abduction (normally, about 90°)
• Circumduction (normally, about 360°, small circle)

Type of joint
• Hinge (thumb only)

Movement
• Flexion (normally, about 90°)
• Extension (normally, thumb is straight in neutral position)

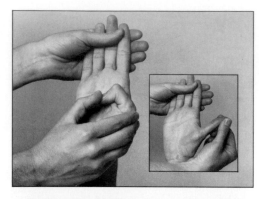

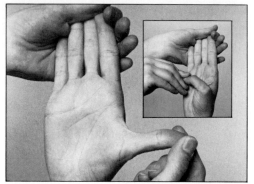

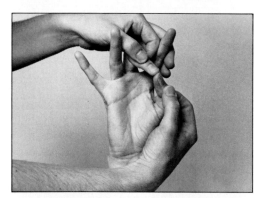

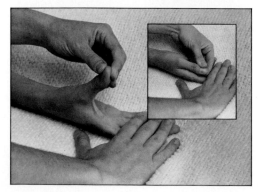

1 To flex and extend the condyloid and hinge joints of your patient's thumbs, position her right upper arm and elbow flat against the bed, with her forearm at a 90° angle to the bed. With your left hand, firmly grasp your patient's right fingers. With your right hand, flex the first two joints of her thumb, as the nurse is doing here.

[Inset] Then, straighten her thumb. Repeat this exercise at least three times.

Follow the same procedure on her left thumb.

2 Next, flex, extend, and hyperflex the saddle joints of your patient's thumbs. With your left hand, firmly grasp your patient's right fingers, making sure her thumb's against her index finger. Then, move her thumb laterally, as shown here.

[Inset] Now, flex her thumb toward her palm. Repeat this exercise at least three times.

Follow the same procedure on her left thumb.

3 Now we'll show you an opposition exercise for your patient's thumbs. First, hold your patient's right index finger with your left hand. Now, with your right hand, touch her right thumb to her index finger. Then, hold her right middle finger, and touch her thumb to it, as shown. Continue touching the thumb to each fingertip. Repeat this exercise at least three times.

Follow the same procedure on her left thumb.

4 Now, adduct and abduct the saddle joints of your patient's thumbs. To do this, place the back of your patient's right hand against the bed. With your left hand, gently pull her thumb straight up, as shown here. Now, push her thumb down beside her index finger (see inset). Repeat this exercise at least three times.

Follow the same procedure on her left thumb.

How to perform range-of-motion (ROM) exercises on your patient's hips

You'll need to guide your patient through nine separate hip movements to correctly perform ROM exercises. Use the chart below for review. Then, read the following photostory for detailed instructions on how to perform each exercise.

An important reminder: If, at any time, your patient feels pain or you meet resistance when performing an exercise, stop immediately.

Caution: Never circumduct your patient's hips unless she can stand on one leg. Circumduction is usually an active or active assistive exercise.

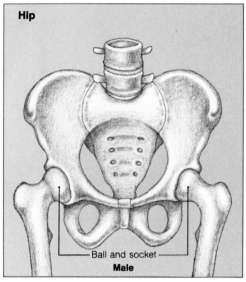

Hip

Ball and socket
Male

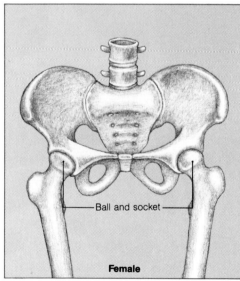

Ball and socket
Female

Type of joint
• Ball and socket

Movement
• Adduction (normally, hip is straight in neutral position)
• Cross adduction (normally, about 45°)
• Abduction (normally, about 65°)
• Internal rotation (normally, about 35°)
• External rotation (normally, about 42°)
• Flexion (normally, about 135°)
• Extension (normally, hip is straight in neutral position)
• Hyperextension (normally, about 42°)
• Circumduction (normally, about 360°)

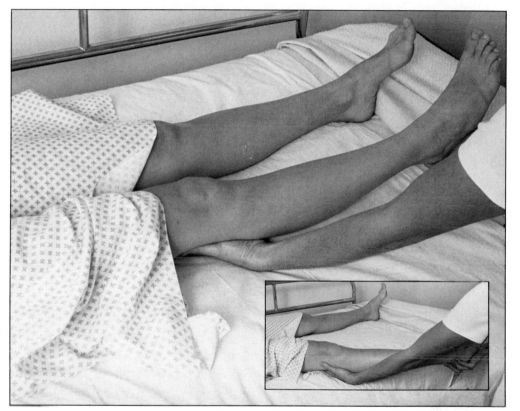

1 This photostory shows you how to adduct and abduct your patient's hip joints. First, place your patient in a supine position. Then, put your left hand under her right knee, and grasp her right heel with your right hand. Next, raise her right leg about 2″ (5 cm).
[Inset] Then, pull her right leg toward you, as the nurse is doing here.

2 Gently move your patient's right leg in the opposite direction, across her left leg (cross adduction).
Important: Check with the doctor before performing this exercise, as it may be contraindicated for some knee and hip disorders. Repeat this exercise at least three times.
Then, follow the same procedure on her left hip.

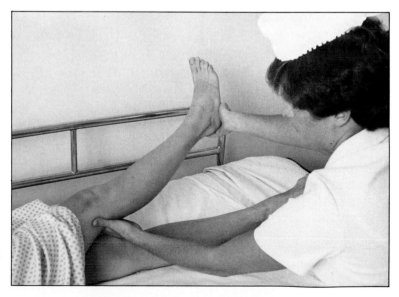

Reviewing exercises

How to perform range-of-motion (ROM) exercises on your patient's hips continued

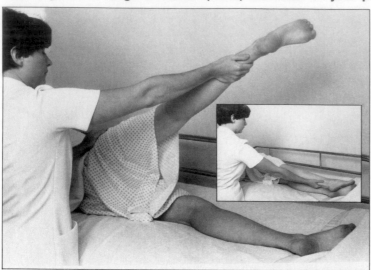

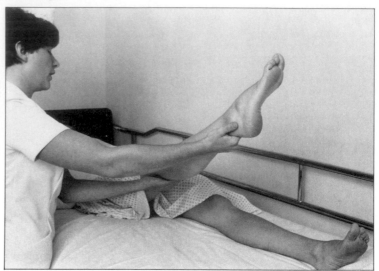

3 If your patient must lie on her side, you can adduct and abduct her hips as follows: Stand facing her back. If she's lying on her left side, place your left hand on her right hip. Support your patient's right calf with your right hand, as shown in this photo. Now, raise her leg as high as possible.

[Inset] Then, lower her leg. Repeat this exercise at least three times.

Follow the same procedure on her left hip.

4 Next, we'll show you internal and external hip rotation exercises. Make sure your patient's on her back, with her legs straight and her toes pointing up. Abduct her right leg. Then, place your left hand on her right thigh and your right hand on her right ankle. Roll her leg toward the body's midline, keeping her knee straight and her leg axis fairly constant.

[Inset] Now, roll her leg toward you. Repeat this exercise at least three times.

Follow the same procedure on her left hip.

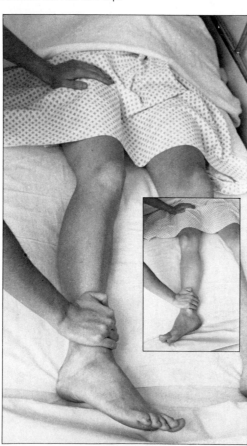

5 Here's a way to flex and extend your patient's hip joints. First, place your patient flat on her back, and support her right knee and heel. Raise her right leg as high as possible, as shown here.

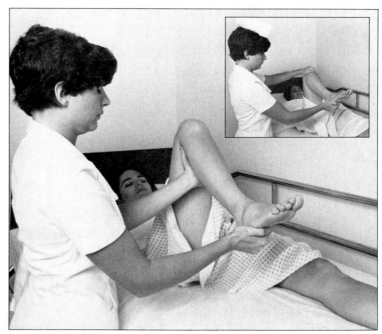

6 Bend your patient's right knee, guiding her thigh toward her chest, as the nurse is doing here.

[Inset] Then, reposition your left hand on top of her right knee. Press her knee toward her chest to flex her hip as much as possible.

Straighten her leg, and lower it to the bed. Repeat this exercise at least three times.

Follow the same procedure on her left hip.

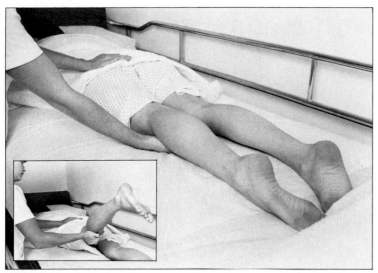

7 To hyperextend her hip joints, place your patient on her abdomen. Then, stand close to her left knee. Place your right hand under her left knee. Place your left hand on her left hip, and apply pressure to stabilize her hip.

[Inset] Next, raise your patient's leg as high as possible. Then, lower it.

Follow the same procedure on her right hip.

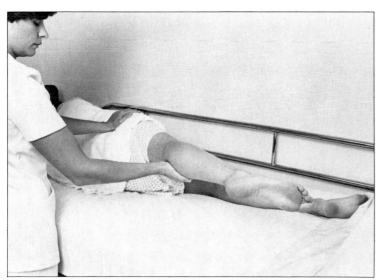

8 Suppose your patient's on her left side. You can also hyperextend her hips in this position by placing your left hand on her right hip. Position your right hand under her right knee. Pull her right leg toward you as far as possible. Then, return it to the starting position.

Follow the same procedure on her left hip.

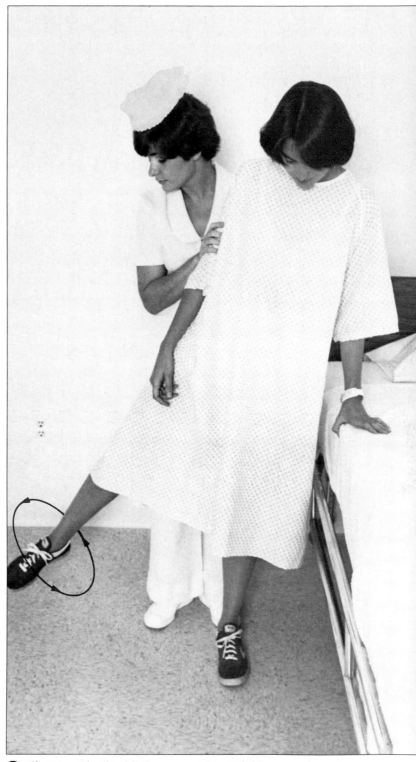

9 If your patient's able to support her weight on one leg, show her how to circumduct her hip joints. Have her stand on her left leg. Tell her to move her right leg in a circle for three complete turns. If she's able, have her stand on her right leg and move her left leg the same way.

Reviewing exercises

How to perform range-of-motion (ROM) exercises on your patient's knees

You'll need to guide your patient through two separate knee movements to correctly perform ROM exercises. Use the chart below for review. Then, read the following photostory for detailed instructions on how to perform each exercise.

An important reminder: If, at any time, your patient feels pain or you meet resistance when performing an exercise, stop immediately.

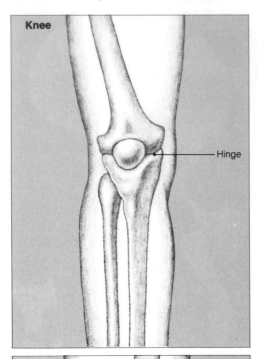

Knee

Hinge

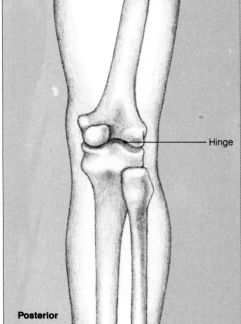

Posterior

Type of joint
• Hinge

Movement
• Flexion (normally, about 142°)
• Extension (normally, knee is straight in neutral position)

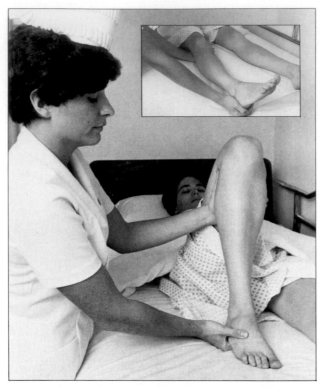

1 Are you ready to flex and extend your patient's knee joints? If so, follow these guidelines: First, position your patient so she's flat on her back. Then, place your left hand under your patient's right knee. Put your right hand under her right heel. Bend your patient's right knee until her heel touches her thigh—or as close to it as possible.
[Inset] Then, straighten her knee. Repeat this exercise at least three times.
Then, follow the same procedure on her left knee.

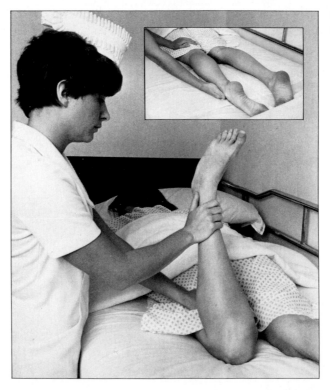

2 If your patient's lying on her abdomen, you can flex and extend her knee joints this way: Place your left hand on your patient's left thigh. Grasp her left ankle with your right hand. Now, bend her knee until her heel touches her buttocks—or as close to them as possible.
[Inset] Then, straighten her knee. Repeat this exercise at least three times.
Follow the same procedure on her right knee.

How to perform range-of-motion (ROM) exercises on your patient's ankles

You'll need to guide your patient through five separate ankle movements to correctly perform ROM exercises. Use the chart below for review. Then, read the following photostory for detailed instructions on how to perform each exercise.

An important reminder: If, at any time, your patient feels pain or you meet resistance when performing an exercise, stop immediately.

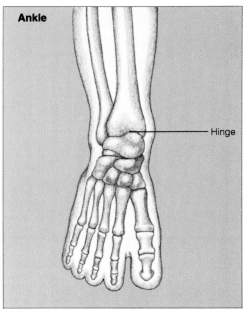

Ankle

Hinge

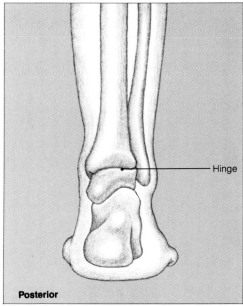

Hinge

Posterior

Type of joint
• Hinge

Movement
• Extension (normally, ankle is straight in neutral position)
• Dorsiflexion (also called flexion; normally, about 10°)
• Plantar flexion (also called hyperextension; normally, about 45°)
• Inversion (normally, about 20°)
• Eversion (normally, about 20°)

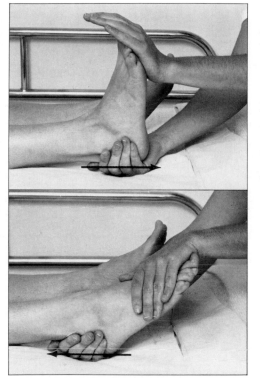

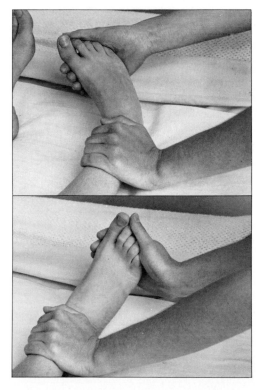

1 Now, we'll explain how to perform dorsiflexion and plantar flexion on your patient's ankles. First, place your patient flat on her back, with her legs straight and her toes pointing up. Support her right heel with your right hand.

Put your left hand on the ball of your patient's right foot. Then, as shown in the top photo, push against her foot as you gently pull on her heel.

[Lower photo] Keeping your right hand under her right heel, place your left hand on *top* of her foot. Push her foot down as you gently push her heel back, as the nurse is doing here. Repeat both exercises at least three times.

Then, follow the same procedure on her left ankle.

2 To perform inversion/eversion exercises on your patient's ankles, follow these instructions: Place your left hand on her right ankle. Grasp her right foot with your right hand, and move her foot to one side.

[Lower photo] Then, move her foot to the other side. Repeat this exercise at least three times.

Follow the same procedure on her left ankle.

Reviewing exercises

How to perform range-of-motion (ROM) exercises on your patient's feet and toes

You'll need to guide your patient through 11 separate foot and toe movements to correctly perform ROM exercises. Use the chart below for review. Then, read the following photostory for detailed instructions on how to perform each exercise.

An important reminder: If, at any time, your patient feels pain or you meet resistance when performing an exercise, stop immediately.

PATIENT TEACHING

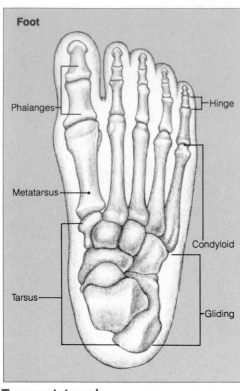

Foot

- Phalanges
- Metatarsus
- Tarsus
- Hinge
- Condyloid
- Gliding

Tarsometatarsal

Type of joint
- Gliding (between tarsals only)

Movement
- Flexion (minimal)
- Extension (minimal)
- Adduction (minimal)
- Abduction (minimal)

Metatarsophalangeal

Type of joint
- Condyloid

Movement
- Flexion (normally, about 45°)
- Extension (normally, toe is straight in neutral position)
- Hyperextension (normally, about 90°)
- Adduction (normally, about 20°)
- Abduction (normally, about 20°)

Type of joint
- Hinge

Movement
- Flexion (normally, about 90°)
- Extension (normally, toe is straight in neutral position)

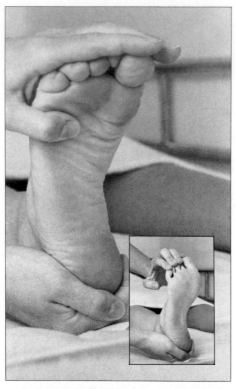

1 Ready to flex and extend your patient's foot and toe joints? First, place her flat on her back, with her legs straight and her toes pointing up. Support her right heel with your right hand. With your left hand, flex her toes down, as shown in this photo.

[Inset] Then, push her toes up. Repeat this exercise at least three times.

Follow the same procedure on her left foot.

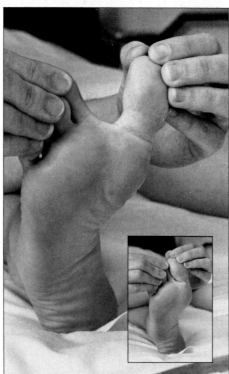

2 Next, you'll want to adduct and abduct your patient's toes. To do this, support your patient's right toes. Move her big toe away from its adjacent toe as far as possible.

[Inset] Now move it back again. Repeat this exercise at least three times. Then, perform this exercise on her other toes.

Follow the same procedure on her left foot.

Performing isometric exercises

The home care aid that follows will help you teach your patient how to perform isometric exercises properly. As you probably know, these exercises will help increase any patient's muscle strength and tone.

Which patients benefit most from isometric exercises? Those who are on complete bed rest. For these patients, you can use isometric exercises to supplement range-of-motion exercises and help them gain confidence by participating actively in their own care.

Before starting a program of isometric exercises with any patient, get the doctor's OK. When you explain the exercises to your patient, remind him to breathe regularly and deeply as he tightens his muscles. (This will prevent him from performing a Valsalva maneuver.)

Finally, give your patient a copy of the home care aid, and review the instructions with him.

Patient teaching

Home care

How to do isometric exercises

Dear Patient:
After you leave the hospital, the doctor wants you to continue the isometric exercises you've learned to help you strengthen and tone your muscles. By performing these exercises regularly, you'll find it easier to carry out your day-to-day activities.

Work this isometric program into your daily routine, repeating each exercise three times and the entire program at least five times a day. Use the following instructions as a guide:

1 First, strengthen your arm muscles. Hold your arms in front of you, with your palms together. As you breathe slowly and deeply, press your hands together firmly, or grasp a ball in each hand, for 3 to 5 seconds. Now relax. Remember, increased arm strength will make it easier for you to transfer, move in bed, or propel a wheelchair.

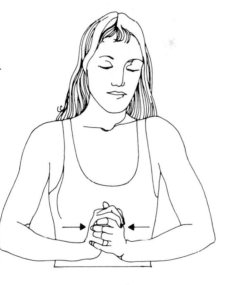

2 Next, strengthen the muscles in your abdomen. To do this, pull your abdominal muscles in as tightly as you can for 3 to 5 seconds. Breathe slowly and deeply. Then, relax the muscles gradually.

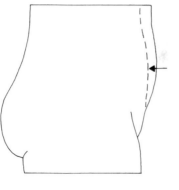

3 Now, exercise the muscles in your buttocks. As you breathe slowly and deeply, tighten your buttocks' muscles for 3 to 5 seconds. Then, relax them. Strengthening these muscles will help you stay balanced when you're seated.

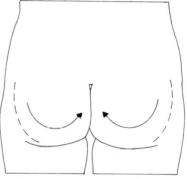

4 Then, strengthen your leg muscles. Lie on your back and bend your left leg at the knee. Keeping your left foot flat on the floor, raise your right leg 3″ (7.6 cm), and hold it there for 5 seconds. Then, lower it. Relax your legs. Repeat the exercise, raising your left leg.

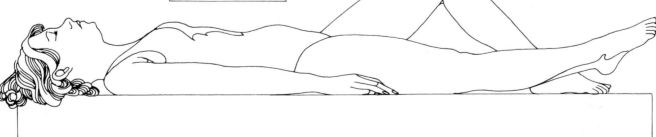

Special considerations

Caring for a patient with a special mobility problem? For example, a patient who's had a leg amputated or a breast removed? In this section, we'll show you some special guidelines and precautions you'll need to know.

We'll tell you:
• how to properly bandage a stump, whether it's above or below the knee.
• how to teach hip abduction exercises to a patient with a leg amputation.
• how to teach strengthening exercises to a patient who's had a mastectomy.
• what to do when your patient's stump has drainage.

In addition, we'll provide you with tips to help you do your job better. Study the following pages carefully.

PATIENT PREPARATION

Patient preparation for a leg amputation
Your patient will be very frightened of having his leg amputated. To begin with, he'll be worried about how the surgery—the loss of his leg—will hamper his life-style. And if he's a child, his fears will be compounded by his limited understanding of surgical procedures. Do your best to help your patient relax. Relieve some of his anxiety by trying to anticipate and answer all his questions. Also, be sure to answer any questions his family and friends may have.

Remember: Depending on the reason for your patient's amputation—for example, severe trauma—you may not have time to thoroughly prepare your patient before surgery. However, try to prepare him as much as possible.

Begin by finding out exactly what your patient expects. Clear up any misconceptions he has about the surgery. Be supportive. Explain:
• why he needs surgery.
• how he'll be prepared for surgery.
• how he'll be cared for after surgery, including his need for pain medication.
• how the loss of his limb may limit his activities.
• what he can do to regain his strength and mobility.

Then, if you know how your patient will be walking after surgery—for example, with crutches, a cane, or a walker—have the physical therapist teach him the appropriate gait. Or, if a physical therapist isn't available, you'll have to teach him. Urge him to practice this gait *before* surgery, if possible, and praise his efforts. Discuss the need to perform range-of-motion exercises after surgery, to increase his joint mobility and strength. Demonstrate the exercises, and encourage him to practice them before surgery, if possible. (For more information on range-of-motion exercises, see pages 46 to 63.)

Teach your patient how he can prevent respiratory complications after surgery by turning, coughing, and deep breathing. Encourage him to practice the correct methods before surgery.

Remember, because your patient is scared, he may forget much of what you've told him. So, after surgery, continue to reinforce these instructions. If the doctor says it's OK, you may want to ask someone who has had a leg amputated to talk with your patient.

Important: If your patient feels uncomfortable talking with you, ask another health-care professional to try to talk with him.

Stump bandaging after an above-the-knee amputation

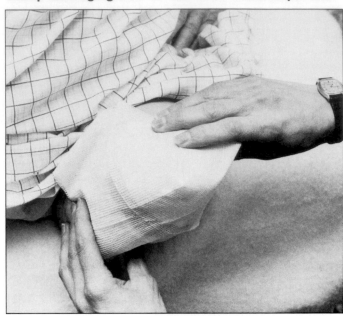

1 *Your patient, 59-year-old Peter Callis, is an uncontrolled diabetic with a varicose ulcer that's not responding to treatment. Several days ago, the doctor amputated Mr. Callis' left leg above his knee. Now the doctor asks you to bandage his stump. Do you know how? If you're unsure, follow these steps:*

First explain to Mr. Callis that the bandaging procedure will help reduce swelling and mold his stump for a prosthesis. Also, tell him you'll teach him the procedure as you perform it. Then place him in low or semi-Fowler's position, or have him sit on the edge of the bed. Wash your hands.

Then, remove the elastic bandage. Obtain a clean 4″ (10.2 cm) elastic bandage. Remove any dressing and discard it. Wash your hands again. Check your patient's leg for signs of circulatory impairment or infection. Notify the doctor if any signs are present. Otherwise, redress the wound.

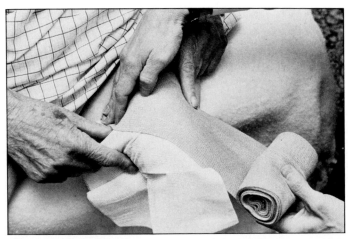

2 Hold the end of the elastic bandage at the top anterior surface of Mr. Callis' leg. Or, ask your patient to hold the bandage, if he can. Then, bring the bandage diagonally downward toward the end of his stump.

3 Applying even pressure, bring the bandage diagonally upward, close to his groin area.

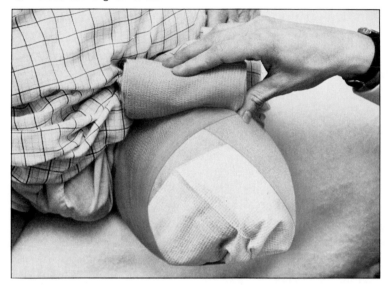

5 Next, bring the bandage diagonally under Mr. Callis' buttocks to the opposite iliac crest, and then diagonally back toward his stump, as shown here.

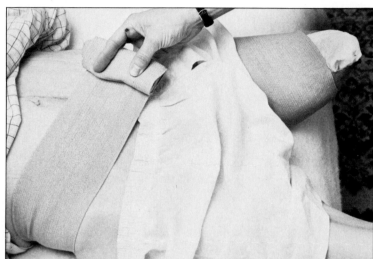

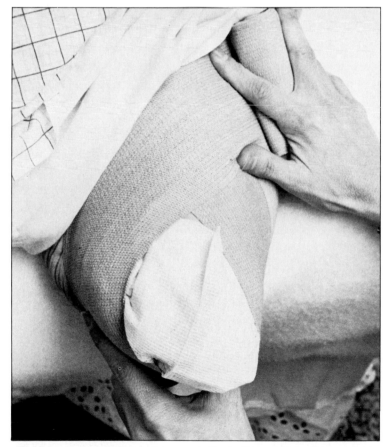

4 Now, secure the bandage end. To do this, make a figure-eight turn with the bandage, wrapping it around the top of your patient's leg, downward under his stump, and back to the groin area, as the nurse is doing here. Then repeat the figure-eight turn two times.

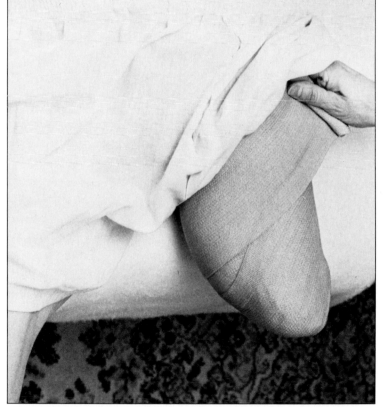

6 Making figure-eight turns, wrap the bandage around your patient's stump until it's completely covered.

Finally secure the bandage with clips, safety pins, or adhesive tape. If you're using clips or safety pins, make sure they're on the stump's anterior side. Doing so prevents possible pressure areas.

Document the rebandaging procedure in your nurses' notes.

Special considerations

Stump bandaging after a below-the-knee amputation

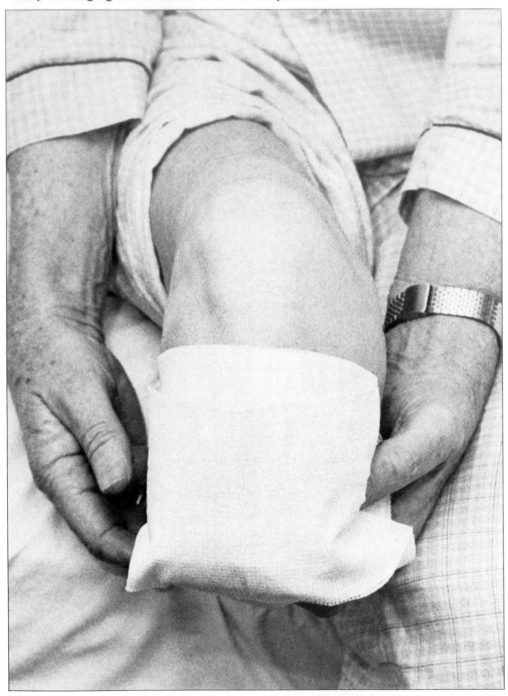

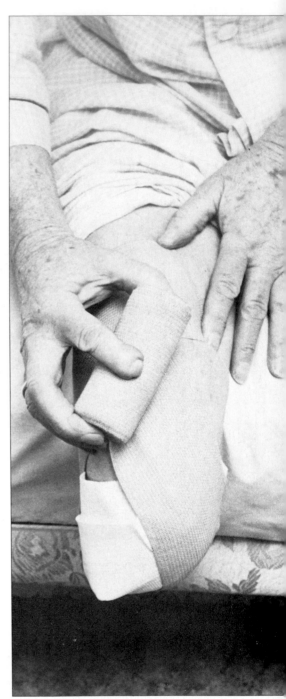

1 *Imagine that 45-year-old Kenneth Moore had his right leg amputated below the knee. You'll need to teach Mr. Moore to properly wrap his stump. Here's how to proceed:*

Begin by explaining to Mr. Moore that rebandaging his stump will help reduce swelling and start molding his stump for a prosthesis. Then, have him sit on the edge of the bed. After you've shown your patient how to wrap the bandage, allow him to practice.

2 First, have Mr. Moore use one hand to hold the end of the elastic bandage just above the bend of his knee. With his other hand, tell him to bring the bandage downward to the distal end of his stump. Remind him to be careful not to fold or crease the elastic bandage.

When he reaches the end of the stump, instruct him to bring the bandage upward in a diagonal direction, as shown here.

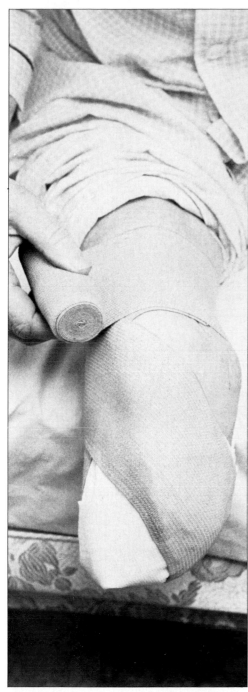

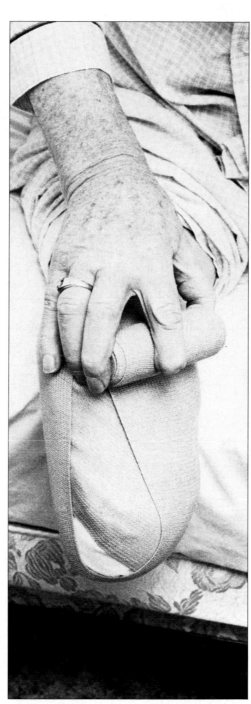

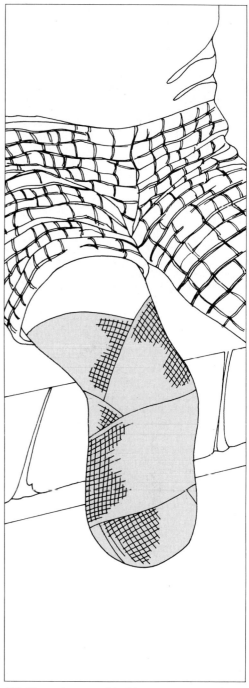

3 Then, have Mr. Moore bring the bandage above his knee to begin making a figure-eight turn. To ensure proper venous blood return, tell your patient to apply less tension on the bandage above the knee than on the end of the stump.

4 Have Mr. Moore continue the figure-eight turn to cover his stump-end and his knee.

5 Then, instruct Mr. Moore to repeat the figure-eight pattern two more times until his stump and knee are completely covered. Have him secure the bandage with clips, safety pins, or adhesive tape.

Document the entire procedure, including your patient teaching, in your nurses' notes.

Special considerations

Amputation: When the patient has a plaster cast

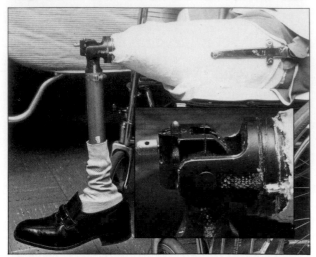

Picture this: Your patient has had his left leg amputated, and the doctor has put a plaster cast on his stump. This will control edema and improve circulation. Such a cast will also permit your patient to walk earlier, because it can be fitted with a temporary prosthesis (see inset). Do you know how to care for your patient in this situation?

Begin by checking his cast for signs of drainage. If you observe any drainage on the cast, circle the area—on the cast—with a felt-tip pen. Note the date and time of your observation next to the circle. Then, document the information in your nurses' notes. Continue to check the circled area frequently for increased drainage or bleeding. If you note a constant increase, notify the doctor immediately.

Check for tightness by slipping two fingers between the cast and your patient's skin. If you can slip more than two fingers into the cast, it may be too loose. If you can't slip your fingers into his cast, suspect bleeding, severe edema, or inflammation. Notify the doctor immediately.

Remember to check the cast for rough edges. If you note any, apply adhesive tape over the edges to petal the cast. Then, look for pressure signs on your patient's skin: for example, blanched or reddened areas. If you observe any, notify the doctor. He may trim the rough areas of the cast or insert extra padding.

Important: If your patient complains of increasing or severe pain at any time, call the doctor immediately.

Strengthening exercises: When your patient has had a leg amputated

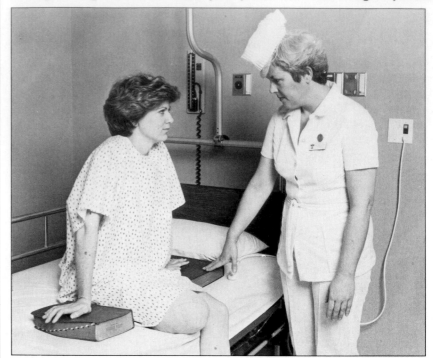

1 *Consider this situation: Ginny Long, a 25-year-old writer, has just had her right leg amputated below the knee. The doctor instructs you to help Ms. Long perform active and active assistive range-of-motion exercises. Do you know how? Follow these guidelines:*

First, explain the procedure to Ms. Long. Tell her that if at any time she feels pain or meets resistance, she should stop the exercises immediately.

Seat Ms. Long upright in bed, so her right stump is at the edge of the bed and her left leg dangles over the side. Stabilize her lower torso by positioning a wooden block or a thick book on each side of her hips. Have her rest her hands on the books, as shown here.

Now, tell Ms. Long to press down on the books and lift her hips. Then, tell her to lower her hips. Instruct her to repeat this exercise at least three times.

Be sure Ms. Long understands how she'll benefit from this exercise. Remind her that if she's going to use a prosthesis, she'll need strong arms to support the extra weight during crutch walking.

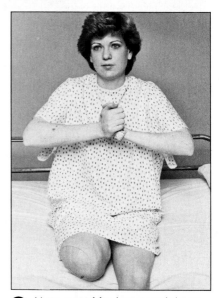

2 Now, seat Ms. Long upright or let her lie down, whichever she prefers. Instruct her to clasp her hands in front of her chest, as shown. Have her push her hands against each other for several seconds, then relax. This exercise helps promote strong arm muscles, which your patient will need when you begin teaching transfer techniques. Tell her to repeat this exercise at least three times.

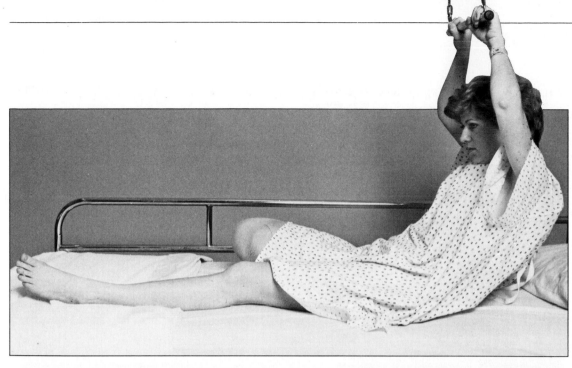

3 Consider asking the doctor to have a trapeze positioned above the bed, so your patient can do some additional arm exercises. For example, by grasping the trapeze bar with both hands, Ms. Long can lift herself to a sitting position. Doing these exercises or position changes helps strengthen her arm muscles and helps prevent decubitus ulcers.

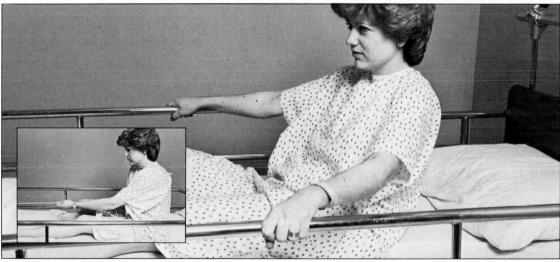

4 Another way your patient can strengthen her arms is by using the bed's side rails to pull herself up in bed.
  Suppose your patient has difficulty using the side rails. Then, attach a nylon rope to the foot of her bed. Tell her to pull herself up, using a hand-over-hand motion, as shown in the inset.

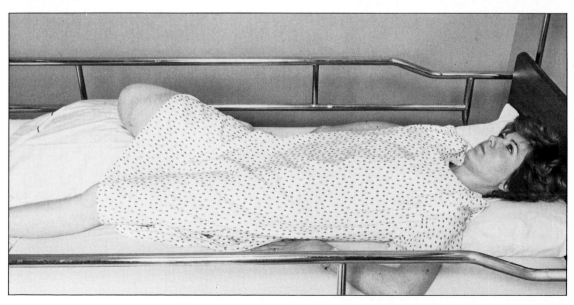

5 Next, place Ms. Long flat on her back. Place pillows under the end of her stump, making sure the stump's higher than her hip. Instruct her to press her stump against the pillows for 2 or 3 seconds, as she attempts to lift her hips off the bed. Have her repeat this exercise at least three times.
  When Ms. Long's finished exercising, remove the pillows, and make sure her hips and knees are fully extended. This helps prevent hip contractures.

Special considerations

Strengthening exercises: When a patient has had a leg amputated continued

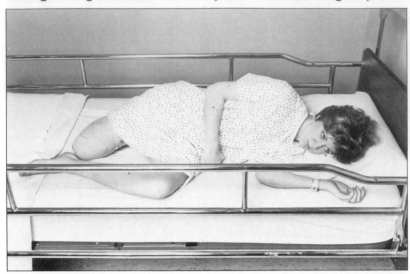

6 Now, position Ms. Long on her left side, so she can perform hip adduction/abduction exercises. Instruct her to flex her left knee and hip forward, as shown here.

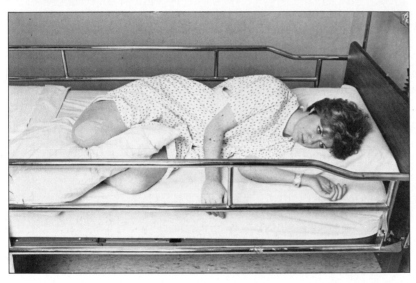

7 Place pillows under her stump, so it's level with her right hip. Have her press her stump against the pillows for 2 or 3 seconds, then stop. Tell her to repeat this exercise at least three times. Remove the pillows after the exercise is completed.

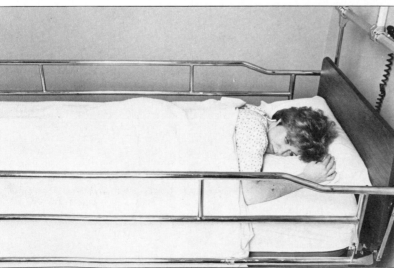

8 After Ms. Long finishes exercising, place her in a prone position for at least 30 minutes. Doing so will ensure that her hips stay fully extended.

PATIENT PREPARATION

Preparing your patient for postmastectomy exercises

Let's assume a patient has just returned to your floor after she has had a mastectomy. Help her increase her strength and mobility by beginning passive range-of-motion exercises within 24 hours or as soon as the doctor says it's OK.

Twice each day—morning and evening—record the amount of edema, if any, in your patient's affected arm. To do this, measure the circumference of the largest part of her forearm, approximately 5″ (12.7 cm) above her wrist.

Also, measure the circumference of the largest part of her upper arm, about 5″ (12.7 cm) above her elbow.

Then, measure the same places on her unaffected arm to establish what's normal.

Nursing tip: For a more accurate measurement of what's normal, measure the affected arm before surgery. Compare and document your findings.

If possible, schedule range-of-motion exercises 30 minutes after your patient receives pain medication. This will minimize some of her discomfort. *But, if she feels severe pain or you meet resistance at any time during the exercises, stop immediately.*

Before you begin, explain the exercise procedure to your patient. Reassure her that you'll be gentle, but tell her to expect some discomfort.

Perform passive range-of-motion exercises on all your patient's joints and extremities until she's able to assist. When you're exercising her affected arm, elevate it on a pillow to prevent edema. Eventually, your patient will do the exercises without assistance (active range-of-motion exercises). When she's achieved normal active exercises, her doctor may want her to start performing active resistive exercises.

Use the steps on the next page as a guideline to performing range-of-motion exercises on your patient's affected arm. Explain each step to her as you do it. Then, when she's ready to be discharged, copy the following home care aid. Fill in all the blanks, and give it to your patient.

Patient teaching

Home care

How to strengthen your muscles after a mastectomy

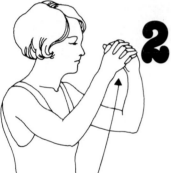

1 Dear Patient:
The nurse has shown you exercises to help strengthen and increase movement in your ____(left/right) arm. Here are some guidelines to help you do the exercises at home. Make sure you perform each exercise at least five times every day.

First, if you can, sit up and clasp your hands in your lap.

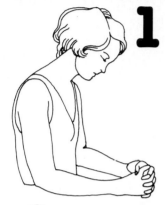

2 With your elbows slightly bent, raise your arms as high as possible. Then, lower them to your lap. Repeat this exercise at least three times.

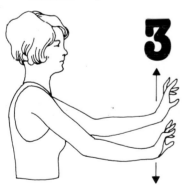

3 When you can, sit or stand facing a wall about 15" (38 cm) away. Walk your fingers up the wall as high as you can. Then, walk your fingers back down. Repeat this exercise at least three times.

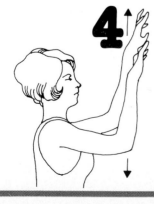

4 After several weeks (or sooner, if possible), gradually move closer to the wall and perform the same exercise. When your toes touch the wall, try extending your arms up the wall as high as you can. Repeat this exercise at least three times.

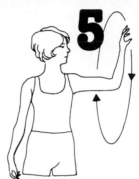

5 Next, turn your body so your ____(left/right) hip and shoulder are about 12" (30.5 cm) from the wall. Walk the fingers of your ____(left/right) hand along the wall in a clockwise motion, as shown here.

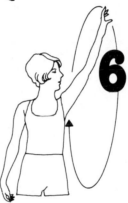

6 After several weeks (or sooner, if possible), gradually move closer to the wall and perform the same exercise. Walk your fingers in a larger circle, keeping your arm straight. Repeat this exercise at least three times.

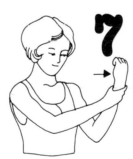

7 Here's how to build muscle strength in your ____ (left/right) arm. Begin by bending this arm at the elbow. With the hand on your other arm, gently straighten this arm as you resist the movement. Repeat this exercise at least three times.

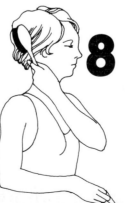

8 Try to increase mobility in your affected arm by using it in your daily activities. For example, exercise your shoulder, elbow, and wrist by brushing your hair, or reaching for items on a shelf.

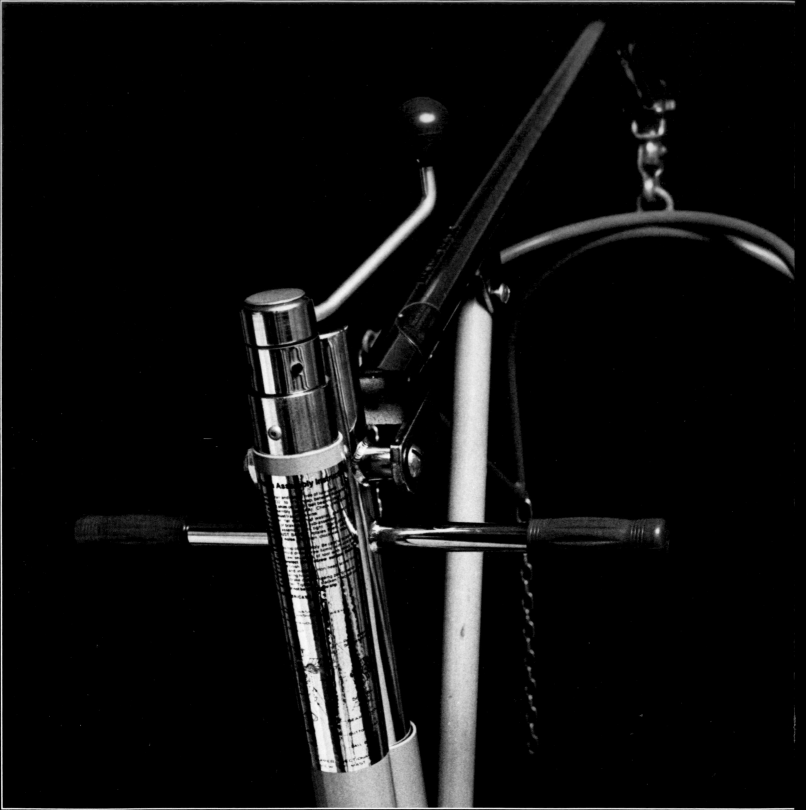

Performing Transfer Techniques

Preparing for transfers

Performing transfers

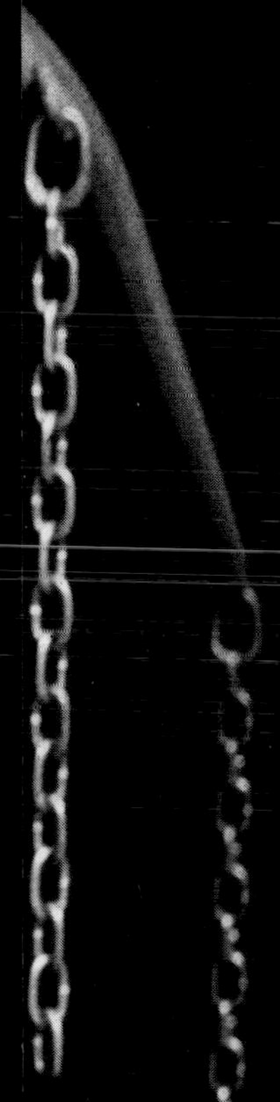

Preparing for transfers

When we talk about transfers we're talking about a variety of different procedures and equipment. For example, depending on your patient's condition, you could need a mechanical lifter or a transfer board to carry out the transfer you've selected. But, all transfers are similar in this respect: they require preparation and evaluation.

Familiarize yourself with the various types of transfer equipment shown on these pages. Then, learn how to use each piece properly.

On the following pages, you'll find out:
• when to use a tub seat.
• when to choose a sitting transfer instead of a standing transfer.
• how to transfer a spinal-injured patient.
• how to evaluate a transfer procedure.

How to select a transfer technique correctly

Are you ready to decide how to transfer your patient? Before selecting a technique, assess your patient's strengths, determine the type and amount of assistance necessary, and familiarize yourself with the available equipment.

To avoid unnecessary risks to yourself and your patient, follow these guidelines:

Assessment

Assessing your patient's strengths and weaknesses should be your first step in selecting a transfer technique. To do this, observe your patient's condition. Note his physical and emotional reaction to increased activity. Look for any joint motion limitations that may affect a transfer.

Also, observe your patient's activities; for example, his ability to move up and down in bed, as well as his ability to turn in bed and sit independently. Determine what your patient can do and how long he can do it.

Observe and evaluate your patient's posture and balance capabilities. For example, when standing, does he lean to one side? Also, check his comprehension and motivation levels. Note his ability to follow your instructions. What's his reaction to increasing his activity level? Is he willing and eager? Or does he seem hesitant?

Then, assess your *knowledge* of your patient's condition. Familiarize yourself with the basics of body mechanics and transfer techniques, so you know the proper way to perform each transfer. Check your own physical strengths and weaknesses. For example, if you have back problems, don't attempt to lift a heavy patient by yourself.

Assistance

Based on your assessment of your patient's physical condition, motivation, comprehension, strength, endurance, and mobility, determine the amount and type of assistance necessary to carry out the transfer. Will you need help? Find out how many coworkers are available.

Equipment

Study the following pages to review the types of transfer equipment available. Familiarize yourself with the equipment in your hospital. Find out how the equipment works, which parts are removable, and how to secure the locks or brakes. Also, find out how to position it properly.

Technique

Next, you're ready to choose the best transfer technique. Decide first whether you want to use a sitting or standing transfer. In most cases, if your patient's able to fully or partially bear weight on one or both legs, you'll perform a *standing* transfer.

But, if your patient's unable to bear weight on one or both legs—for example, a patient with a bilateral amputation—you'll choose a *sitting* transfer.

Learning about transfer equipment

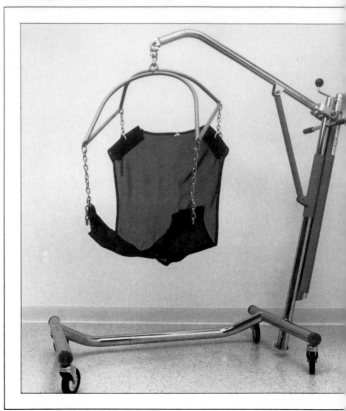

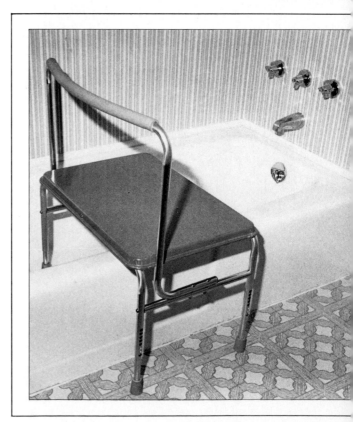

Type
Trans-Aid® mechanical lifter

Description
Canvas or nylon sling seat attached to a metal frame with wheels.

Indication
For a patient who is too heavy or dependent to lift by yourself. Usually used when other methods of transfer are not possible.

Nursing considerations
• Before using, familiarize yourself with the type of lifter used by your hospital. Then, explain and demonstrate the lifter to your patient before proceeding.
• Patient may be showered or immersed in the tub while seated in the sling seat.

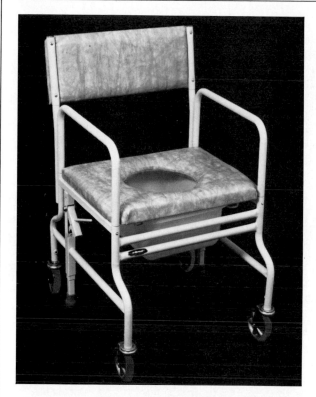

Type
ACTIVEaid® commode chair

Description
Wooden, metal, plastic, or aluminum chair, with a large opening in the center of the seat. Some commodes have bedpans or buckets that slide underneath the opening; other commodes slide directly over the toilet.

Indication
For a patient who can't use a toilet because of physical limitations or architectural barriers.

Nursing considerations
• If chair has wheels, secure brakes or wheel locks before use. Block wheels with sandbags, if necessary.
• Support patient's feet on a footrest or stool.

Type
Tub seat

Description
A wooden, aluminum, or metal bench or stool, with detachable back. Positioned on or over a bathtub.

Indication
For a patient who can perform a sitting transfer but has difficulty lowering himself into a bathtub.

Nursing considerations
• If your patient has poor balance, attach the back to the seat for added support.
• To prevent burns, fill tub and test water temperature before you place patient on seat.
• If you're using a stool, choose one with four legs for a wider support base.
• As your patient's mobility increases, choose a lower bench or stool, so your patient's closer to the water. *Important:* To prevent accidents, make sure the tub you use has handrails and a nonslip surface.

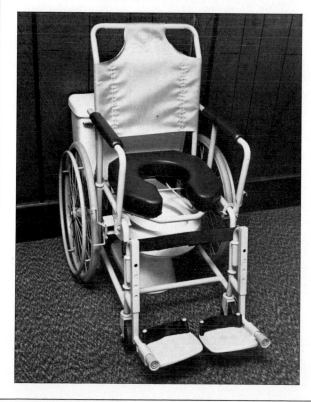

Type
Shower seat

Description
Wooden, aluminum, metal, canvas, or plastic chair or stool. Placed in a shower stall. Some models can also be positioned over a toilet.

Indication
For a patient who can perform a sitting transfer but can't stand long enough to take a shower.

Nursing considerations
• Before transferring patient from wheelchair, adjust shower seat so it's at the same level as the wheelchair seat, if possible.
• If shower seat has wheels, secure brakes or wheel locks before use. Block wheels with plastic-covered sandbags, if necessary.
• If shower seat doesn't have wheels, put rubber tips on the legs of the seat to keep it from moving.
• If your patient has poor balance, make sure the shower seat has a back. Fasten him in the chair with a safety strap. Position his feet on a footrest or stool.
• To prevent burns, adjust water temperature before you transfer patient from wheelchair to shower seat.

Preparing for transfers

Learning about transfer equipment continued

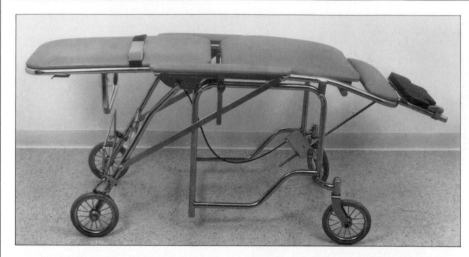

Type
Trans-Aid® Medi-Chair (Stretcher)

Description
Litter with wheels

Indication
For transporting a patient who can't sit in a wheelchair for any reason. Especially useful for postop patients who can't assist with transfer.

Nursing considerations
• Move stretcher close to bed. Lower side rails of bed and stretcher, if any.
• Secure brakes or locks on stretcher wheels.
• Raise side rails on stretcher, and secure patient with safety straps. Transfer patient.
• If stretcher doesn't have safety straps, wrap a rolled sheet around your patient and the stretcher. Be sure to tie it securely.

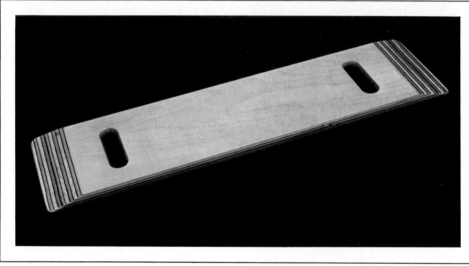

Type
Transfer board

Description
Smooth-surfaced wooden or plastic board approximately 10″ x 24″ (25 x 61 cm). Usually constructed with rounded edges and two hand grips.

Indication
For a patient who is partially or totally dependent; for example, a patient with a spinal injury, hemiplegia, or a bilateral amputation.

Nursing considerations
• Use a board only when both transfer surfaces are at approximately the same height.
• Make sure both ends of the board are positioned securely between transfer surfaces.
• To make the transfer easier, place a drawsheet or disposable pad between your patient and the board.

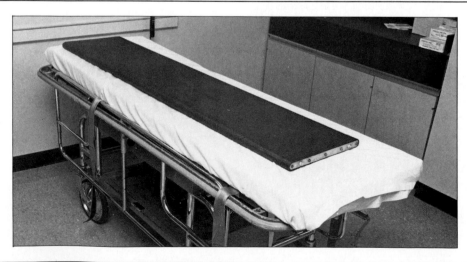

Type
Patient roller board

Description
Canvas or vinyl conveyor belt over aluminum or metal rollers, 2½″ x 5″ (6.3 x 12.7 cm) long, with a fiberglass frame.

Indication
For a patient who must remain in a supine position at all times, except patients who have had back surgery.

Nursing considerations
• Keeps patient's body properly aligned during transfer. Cover the board with sheet before use.

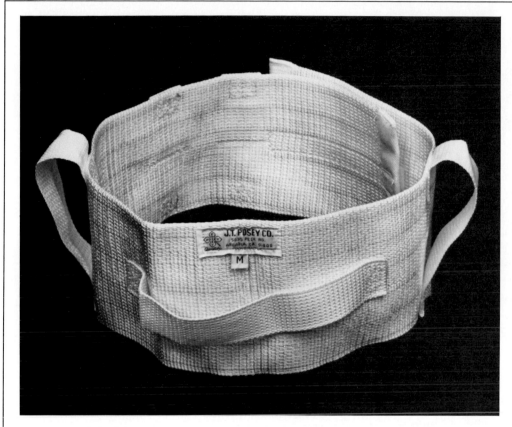

Type
Posey™ Transfer belt (walking belt)

Description
A nylon, canvas, or leather strap about 33″ to 45″ (84 to 114 cm) long, with handles on the sides and back. Usually secured in front with metal buckles.

Indication
For a patient with weakness, dizziness, or poor balance. Also useful when teaching a patient how to walk with crutches, a cane, or a walker. In addition, use when transferring a patient.

Nursing considerations
• When performing transfers, wrap the belt around your patient's waist, over his gown or robe. Fasten it.
• Check for tightness by slipping your fingers between the belt and your patient's waist. Grip the belt to support his balance during transfers, when he's walking, or when you're teaching crutch-walking.

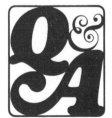

Evaluating the transfer technique
Just as you continually assess and evaluate your patient, you'll assess and evaluate the transfer technique you use. Do you know how to evaluate a technique's effectiveness? If you're unsure, ask yourself these questions:
• Did I select the proper transfer technique? Perhaps not, if you chose a three-person lift and found out your patient was able to roll himself over to the stretcher.
    To avoid choosing the wrong technique, reassess your patient's strengths and weaknesses on a daily basis. Discuss his condition with the doctor and physical therapist (if he has one). Find out which transfer techniques your patient has already learned or is learning.
• Did I use proper body mechanics? If your back hurts after a transfer, you may want to reassess your posture and lifting techniques. (See pages 13 to 17 for details.)
• Did I select the proper equipment? For example, if your patient has spasticity, and you couldn't support him on the transfer board, you may need to use a mechanical lifter.

• How safely and easily was the transfer performed? For example, if your patient couldn't stand steadily during a stand-pivot transfer, you may want to select a transfer board. However, remember that any patient will probably be a little shaky the first time. Check with the doctor or physical therapist. Maybe they can suggest some additional strengthening exercises for your patient.
• How comfortable was my patient during the transfer? Ask your patient. If he had pain or weakness, you may want to see that he gets pain medication before the transfer, or choose another technique. But before you change the technique, check with the doctor and physical therapist to see what could have caused your patient's discomfort.
    Reevaluate your choice of transfer techniques periodically. Then, either continue or revise the technique accordingly. Document in your notes the technique and any changes you make.

Performing transfers

As you know, you'll use a transfer technique or mechanical lifter to move your patient from one area to another. But how well do you understand transfers? For example, do you know:

• when to use a mechanical lifter instead of a transfer technique?

• how to transfer a patient with halo traction?

• what transfer technique to use when your patient can't bear weight on his legs; for example, a patient with bilateral leg amputation?

• how to use a transfer board to move a patient into a car?

• when to use a patient roller board?

• how to teach your patient to perform a standing or sitting transfer?

On these pages, you'll find step-by-step instructions for specific transfer techniques, including the procedures used with a mechanical lifter. We'll explain the reason why you use each one. Read these pages thoroughly to learn how to perform transfers safely.

How to use the three-person lift

1 *Laura Cantor, a 30-year-old executive, has just been transferred to your unit. Ms. Cantor's unconscious after a serious auto accident. You'll use a three-person lift to move her from a stretcher to a bed.*

Before you begin, ask two coworkers to help. But remember, if your patient's obese, you may need three or more co-workers to assist you.

Next, explain the procedure to your patient, even though she's unconscious. Then, loosen the sheet on the stretcher. Make sure your patient's lying supine, with her body well aligned, close to the right side of the stretcher.

Now, position the stretcher at the left side of the bed, as shown here. Make sure the bed's wheels and the stretcher's wheels are locked. Then, adjust the bed to stretcher level. Lower the side rails on the bed and the stretcher. Unfasten the stretcher's safety strap.

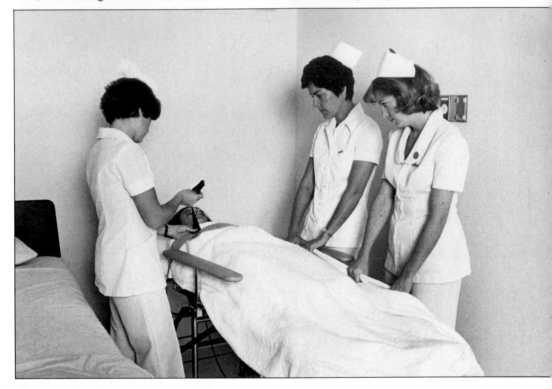

2 Ask the tallest coworker to stand by the left side of the stretcher. (Or, if the stretcher's wide enough, she can kneel on it with her knees apart.) Instruct her to do the following: roll the sheet close to the patient's side; then grasp the sheet with her right hand near the patient's neck and her left hand near the patient's hip.

Ask the other coworker to stand at the foot of the stretcher. Instruct her to support your patient's legs and feet, as the nurse is doing here.

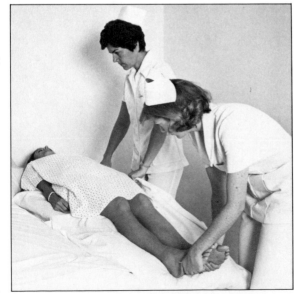

3 Next, kneel in the center of the bed, facing the patient. (Or, if you prefer, you can stand at the right side of the bed.) Spread your knees apart for proper support. Lean over the bed, and roll the sheet close to your patient's side. Grasp the rolled sheet with your left hand near your patient's neck and your right hand near her hip.

If your patient's obese, ask a fourth coworker to position herself on your patient's right side and assist you. You'll support your patient's chest and head; your coworker will support your patient's hips and legs.

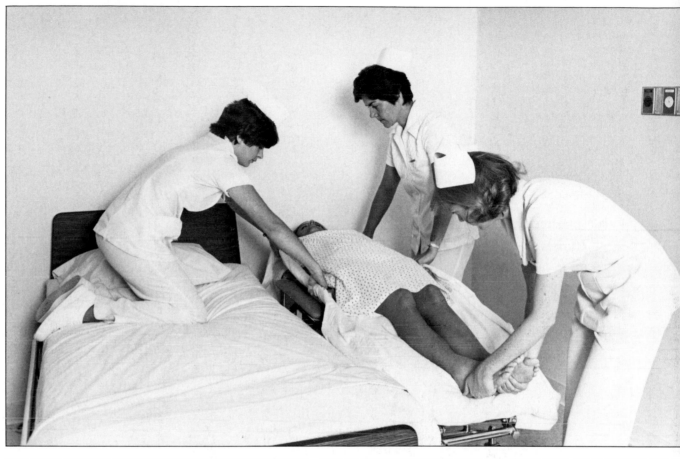

4 On a predetermined signal, slowly lift your patient over to the center of the bed. If your patient's conscious, instruct her to lift her head during the transfer.

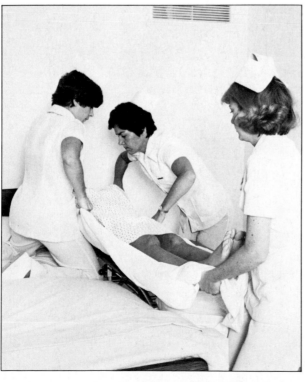

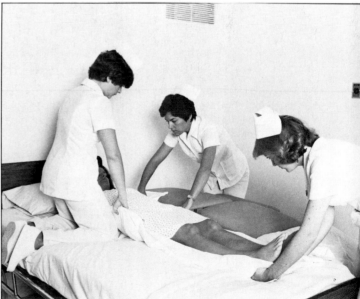

5 Carefully lower your patient onto the bed, keeping her body aligned. When you complete the procedure, raise the bed's side rails.

Remember: You'll reverse the entire procedure to lift your patient back to the stretcher.

Performing transfers

Transferring your patient from a bed to a stretcher

1 *Imagine you want to transfer 24-year-old John Van Pelt from his bed to a stretcher in preparation for surgery. Even though he's drowsy from preop medication, he can still follow instructions. Follow this procedure to make his transfer to the stretcher easier for both of you.*

Begin by explaining the procedure to your patient and reassuring him. Now, lower the bed's left side rail. Position your patient approximately 24″ (61 cm) from the left side of the bed. (If necessary, use a drawsheet to move him, as explained on page 31.)

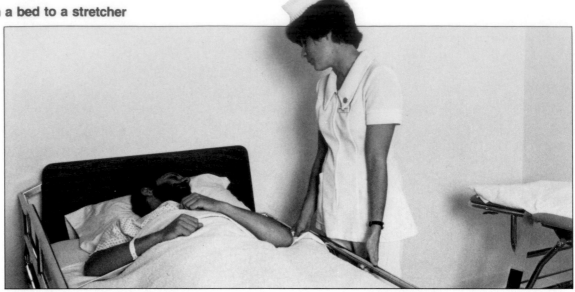

2 Next, position the stretcher lengthwise along the left side of the bed. Lock the wheels of the stretcher and the bed.

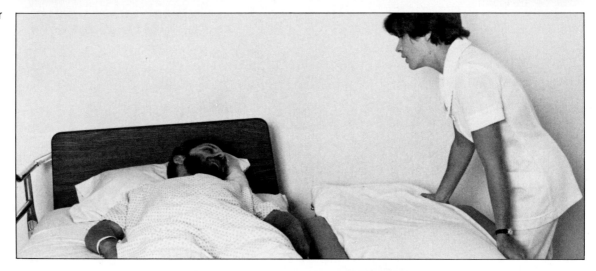

3 Insert pillows or blankets between the bed and the stretcher to create a level surface. Then, stand on the left side of the stretcher to prevent it from moving.

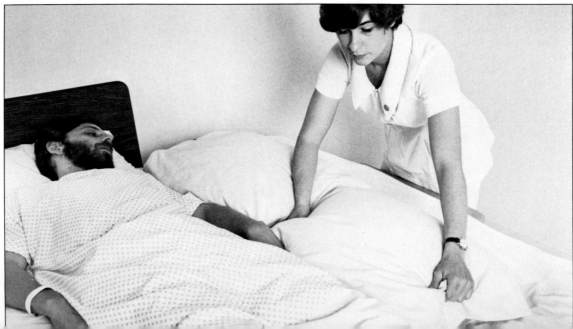

4 If his condition permits, instruct your patient to roll toward his left until he's lying on his stomach. Assist him, if necessary, making sure his body stays well aligned.

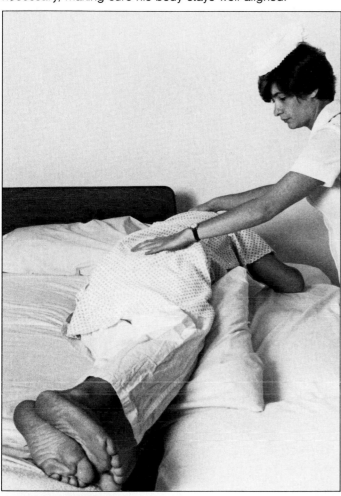

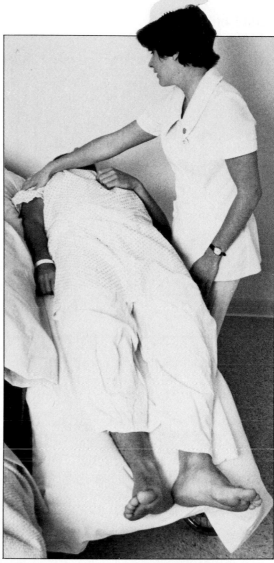

5 Now, tell your patient to continue to roll to his left until he's lying on his back—on the stretcher. Check carefully to make sure his body's well aligned and he's lying in the center of the stretcher.

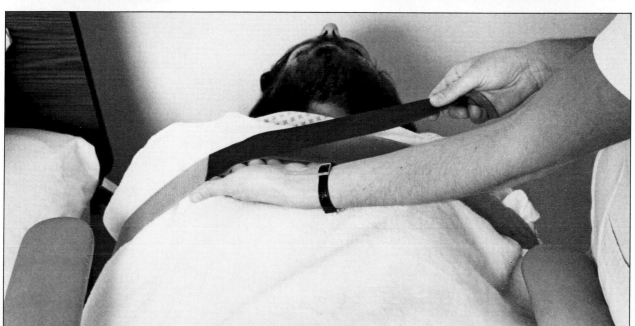

6 Raise the stretcher's side rails. If the stretcher has safety straps, fasten them.
   Document the procedure in your nurses' notes.

Performing transfers

Using the two-person lift technique

1 *Want to transfer 32-year-old Jo Rush from a bed to a wheelchair? Because Ms. Rush is extremely weak, with severe muscle spasms, you decide to use a two-person lift to move her. If you're unsure how to perform this type of transfer, follow these guidelines:*

Before beginning, ask a coworker to help you. But, if your patient's heavy, get two or more coworkers to assist you.

Next, explain the lifting procedure to your patient and reassure her. Then, keeping her body well aligned, use a drawsheet to move her to the left side of the bed (see pages 32 and 33).

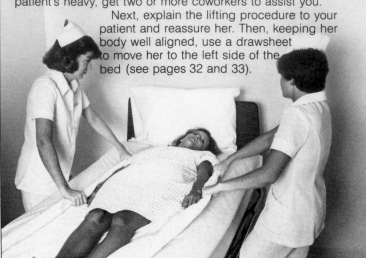

2 Then, move the right side of the wheelchair parallel to the left side of the bed. Lock the wheels on the chair and the bed. Remove the wheelchair's right armrest and both legrests, if possible. If you can't remove the legrests, move them out of the way.

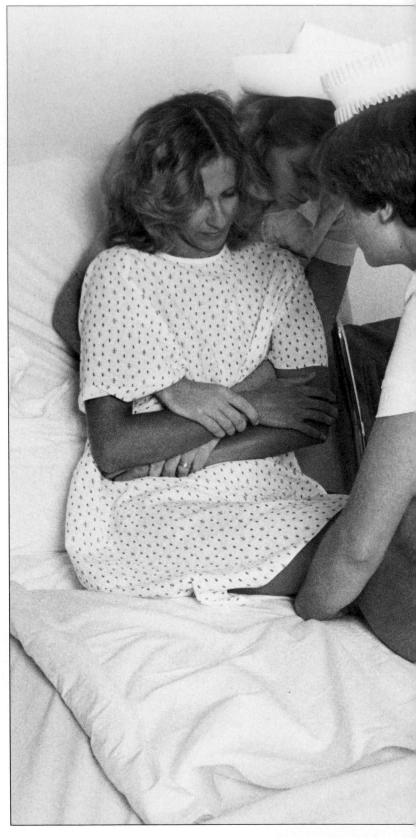

3 Now, raise the bed so it's slightly higher than the wheelchair seat (or slightly higher than the armrests, if they're not removable). To make things easier, you may also want to raise the head of the bed.

Cross your patient's arms over her chest.

[Inset] Now, you and your coworker should position yourselves so the tallest health-care professional is behind the wheelchair. Instruct her to slide her arms under the patient's axillae and firmly grasp her wrists.

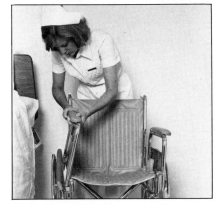

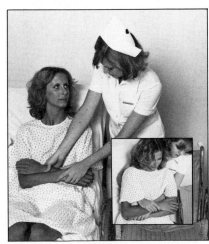

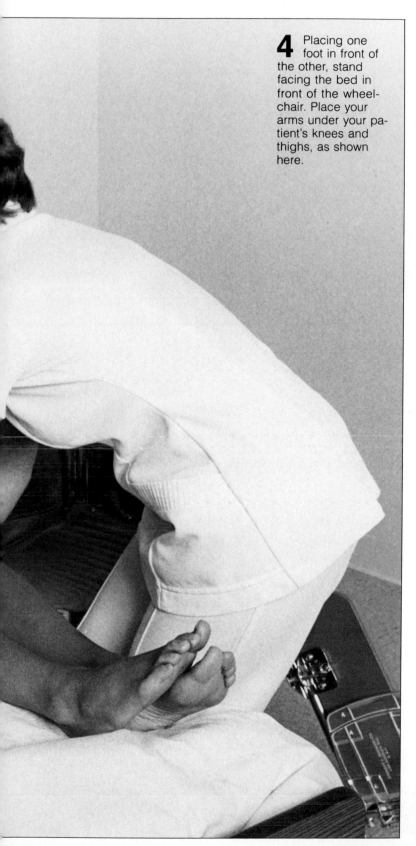

4 Placing one foot in front of the other, stand facing the bed in front of the wheelchair. Place your arms under your patient's knees and thighs, as shown here.

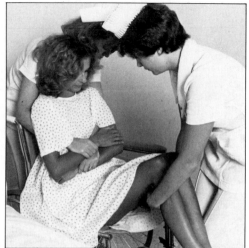

5 Now, at a predetermined signal, lift your patient and pivot toward the wheelchair, as shown here. Slowly lower her into the wheelchair.

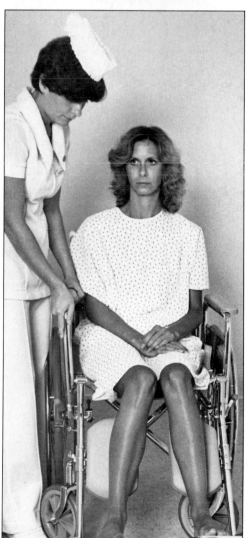

6 Replace the right armrest, and attach or reposition both legrests. Adjust your patient's position, if necessary.
  Reverse the entire procedure to return your patient to her bed.

Performing transfers

How to use the stand-pivot technique to transfer your patient from a bed to a wheelchair

1 *You're about to transfer 56-year-old Frank Shepard, who has left-sided hemiplegia as the result of a cerebrovascular accident (CVA). His care plan indicates that the physical therapist has been teaching him the stand-pivot transfer. Now, you want to show Mrs. Shepard how to help her husband perform this transfer. Do you know how to proceed? Follow these guidelines:*

Begin reviewing the procedure with Mr. and Mrs. Shepard. Emphasize that the transfer can be performed easily at home. Have Mrs. Shepard watch as you help her husband perform the transfer.

First, lower the left side rail. Position the left side of the wheelchair next to the left side of the bed.

Note: Always position the wheelchair on the patient's unaffected side, if possible.

[Inset] Lock the wheels on the chair and the bed. If possible, detach the chair's legrests. Or, move them out of the way.

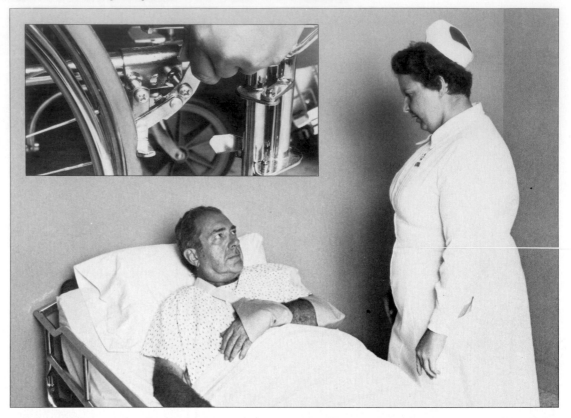

2 Seat Mr. Shepard on the edge of the bed, with his legs hanging over the side. Allow him time to regain his equilibrium. Put shoes on his feet, and be sure his feet are touching the floor. If they aren't, lower the bed.

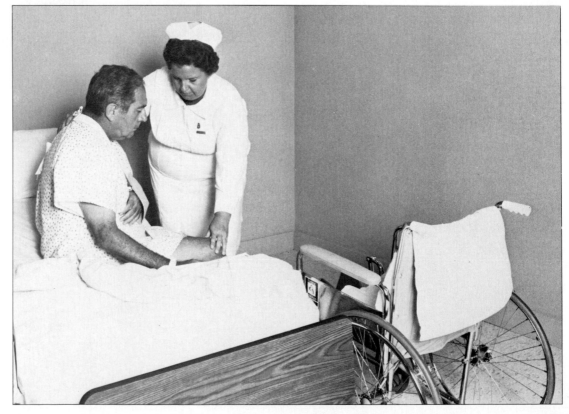

3 Now, move close to Mr. Shepard and place your knees against his knees, as shown here. Squat slightly and slide your arms under his arms. Then, lock your arms around his waist. Be sure to encourage your patient to help as much as possible.

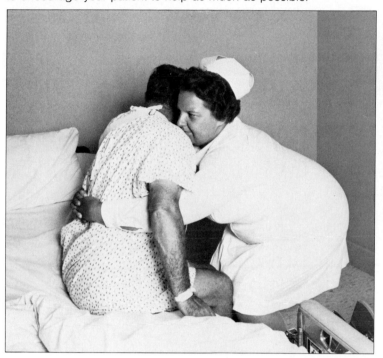

5. Now, have Mr. Shepard grasp the wheelchair's right armrest with his right hand.

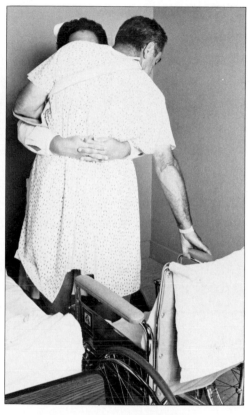

4 Next, instruct Mr. Shepard to use his unaffected arm and leg to push himself up to a standing position. Push your knees against his to keep them stable. Again, allow him a few seconds to regain his equilibrium.

Now, pivot toward the wheelchair, as shown in this photo. Continue to support his knees with your knees as you help him turn his back toward the chair. Stop turning when your patient's back is directly in front of the wheel-chair.

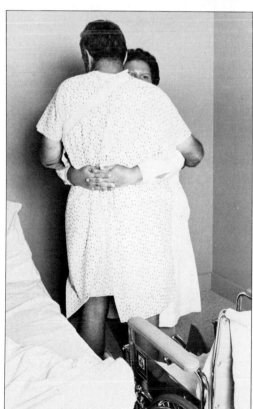

6 Then, as you squat down to lower him into the chair, he'll be able to guide himself into the seat.

Now, explain to Mrs. Shepard how she can arrange to rent or borrow a properly equipped wheelchair for home use. Remember to tell her that the hospital's social service department may be able to help her obtain one, but tell her that it may require a doctor's order.

Finally, document the procedure and any patient teaching in your nurses' notes.

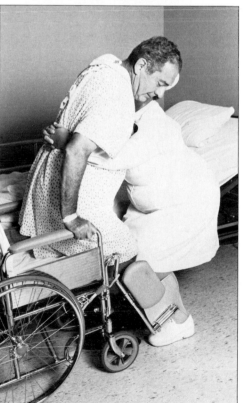

Performing transfers

Transferring your patient from a wheelchair to a car using the stand-pivot technique

1 *Consider this: The doctor has discharged Margaret McKenna and you're asked to transfer her from a wheelchair into a car. Do you know how? Follow these steps carefully:*

Before you begin, thoroughly explain the procedure to your patient and reassure her. If possible, let family members help, because they'll transfer your patient *out* of the car.

Put a transfer belt around your patient's waist. Next, have someone park the car on a level surface, close to the door of the building. Make sure there's enough room for the wheelchair on the right side of the car.

Now, open the car's front passenger door as far as possible. Move the wheelchair over to the car, and if possible, remove the wheelchair's left armrest and both legrests. (If you can't detach the legrests, move them out of the way.) Then, position the left side of the wheelchair next to the car seat, as shown here. Lock the wheelchair's wheels.

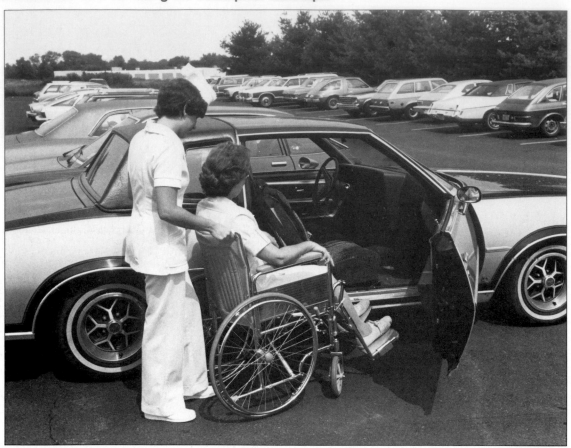

2 Now, follow the procedure explained on page 82 to help your patient to a standing position. Remember to support her knees with your knees throughout the transfer.

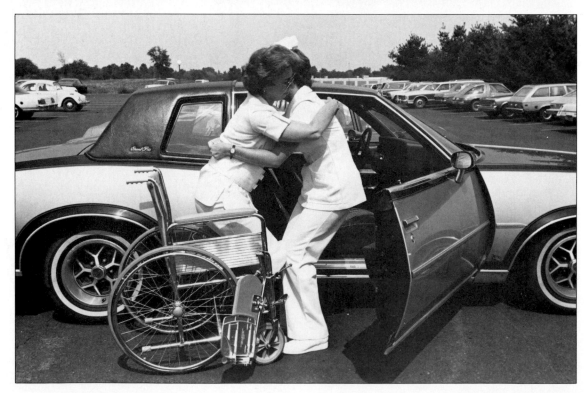

3 Then, pivot toward the car seat, as shown in this photo. Stop turning when your patient's standing directly in front of the open door.

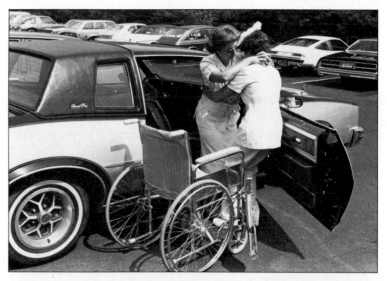

4 Next, slowly lower Ms. McKenna onto the car seat. As you do, make sure her head clears the car's roof. When you've completed this part of the procedure, she'll be sitting with her legs dangling outside the car.

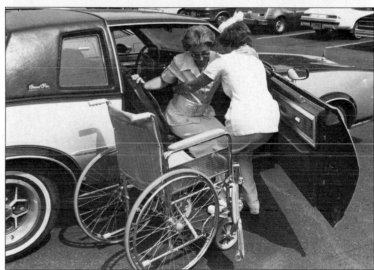

5 Place your hands under your patient's knees and raise her legs into the car. Ask her to help you, if possible, by guiding herself with her arms. Now, make sure she's properly positioned on the car seat, and remove the transfer belt. Finally, fasten her seat belt and close the door.

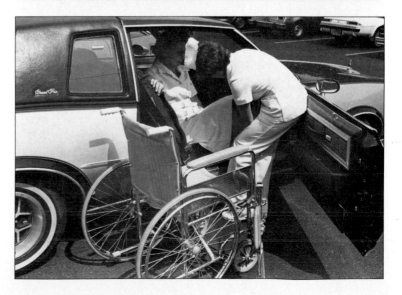

Performing transfers

Standing transfer: How to teach your patient to move from a bed to a wheelchair

1 *Let's say you want to teach 23-year-old Sarah Kowalski how to move herself from a bed to a wheelchair. Because Ms. Kowalski has a weak right side, proceed as follows:*

Begin by explaining the procedure. Then, tell your patient to sit at the edge of the bed, with her feet flat on the floor. Make sure she's wearing shoes. If the bed's too high, have her lower it (or lower it for her) until her feet are on the floor.

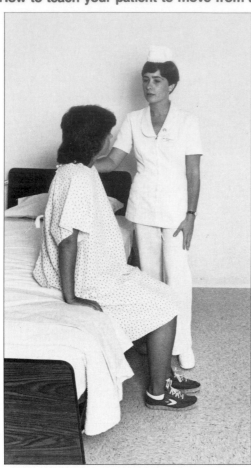

3 Have Ms. Kowalski put her left foot slightly in front of her right foot. Then, instruct her to place her hands, palms down, on the bed, next to her hips.

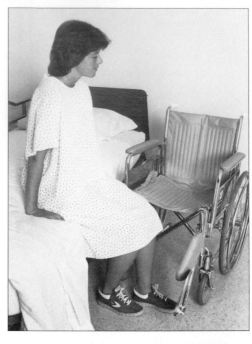

2 Tell your patient to make sure the wheelchair's positioned at a 45° angle to her left side. If she can, have her lock the chair's wheels and move the legrests out of the way.

Or, position the wheelchair for her, and move the legrests out of the way.

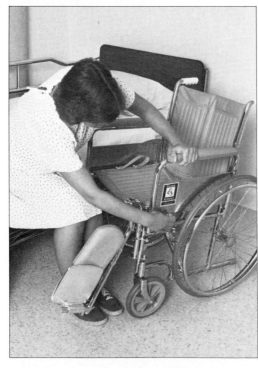

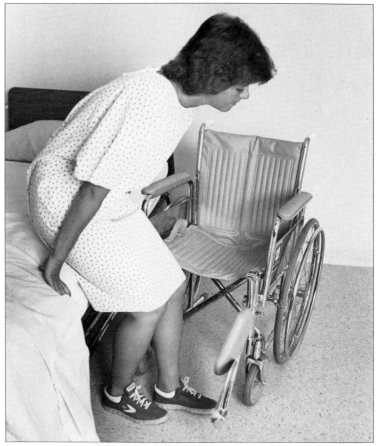

4 Next, ask your patient to lean slightly forward. Tell her to push her hands down on the bed to lift herself to a standing position.

5 Tell your patient to use her left hand to grasp the wheelchair armrest that's farthest from her.

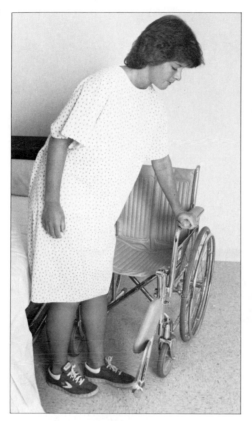

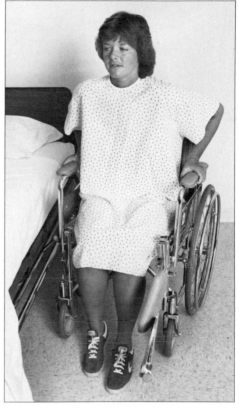

7 Instruct her to support her weight with her hands as she lowers herself into the chair.

6 Then, tell Ms. Kowalski to pivot, or step, to her left, as she grasps the wheelchair's other armrest with her right hand.

Now, ask your patient to position herself directly in front of the wheelchair's seat. The backs of her legs should be touching the edge of the seat.

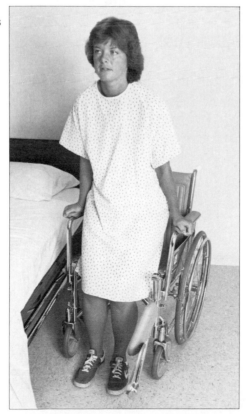

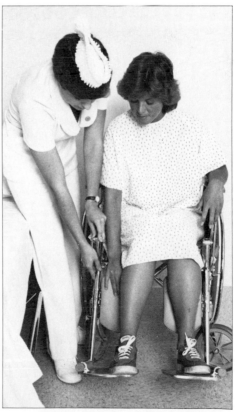

8 Have your patient replace the legrests and position herself in the chair properly. If necessary, replace the legrests for her.

Finally, remind your patient always to keep her wheelchair close to her bed. By doing this she'll have easy access to it. Tell Ms. Kowalski to reverse the procedure to return to the bed.

Performing transfers

Sitting transfer: How to teach your patient to move from a bed to a wheelchair

1 *What if the doctor asks you to teach 33-year-old Janell Marshall how to move herself from a bed to a wheelchair? After checking Ms. Marshall's chart, you see she's recovering from Guillain-Barré syndrome. Do you know how to teach her to perform a sitting transfer? If you're unsure, follow these steps:*

First, explain the procedure to Ms. Marshall, and make sure she's wearing shoes. Then, instruct her to sit at the edge of the bed, with her legs over the side. Her feet should be flat on the floor. Lower the bed, if necessary.

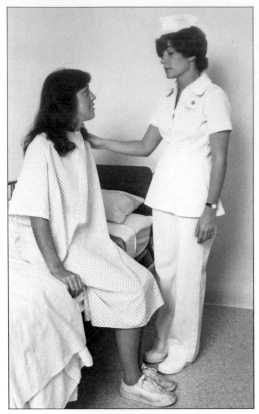

2 Now, tell your patient to move the wheelchair so its right side is parallel to the left side of the bed. Have her lock the wheels.

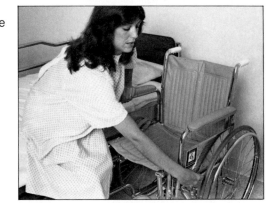

3 Next, ask Ms. Marshall to remove the chair's right armrest. Have her hang the armrest from the side of the chair, as shown here. Then, tell her to remove the right legrest.

Or, remove the armrest and legrest for her.

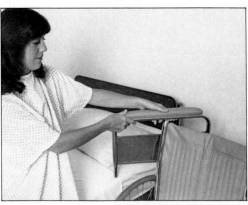
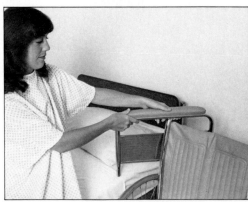

4 Now, instruct your patient to place her left hand, palm down, on the wheelchair seat. Tell her to place her right hand, palm down, next to her right hip, as shown in this photo.

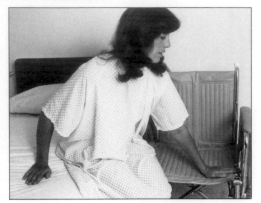

5 Have your patient push down with her right hand, to lift her buttocks off the bed.

Then, tell her to shift her weight to her left hand as she slowly moves herself into the wheelchair seat.

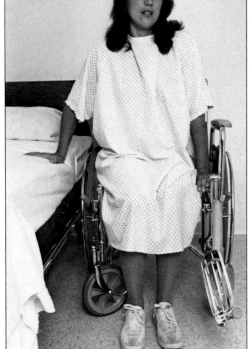

6 Finally, remind Ms. Marshall to reattach the right armrest and legrest. Tell her to position herself properly in the chair.

Have your patient reverse this procedure to return to her bed.

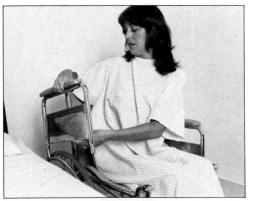
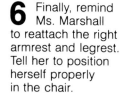

Patient teaching

Home care

How to perform a forward-backward sitting transfer

1 Dear Patient:
Before you leave the hospital, your doctor wants you to learn how to get from your bed to your wheelchair. To learn how to do this transfer, follow these guidelines:

First, remove the wheelchair's legrests. If they're not removable, swing them aside. Then, position the front of the wheelchair as close as possible to the side of the bed. Lock its wheels. If you can't position the wheelchair yourself, ask someone to do it for you. The seat of the wheelchair should be facing the side of the bed.

Make sure you're sitting in bed with your legs extended.

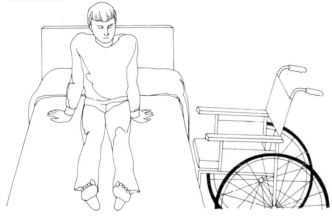

2 Next, lean slightly forward. Pushing your hands against the mattress, lift your buttocks slightly off the bed. Keeping your legs extended across the bed, inch backward to the side of the bed—close to the wheelchair. Stop when your back is directly in front of the wheelchair.

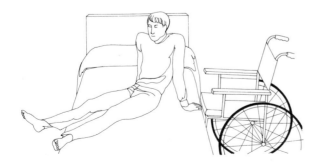

3 Now, firmly grasp the armrests of the wheelchair, and gradually lift your buttocks onto the seat. Unlock the wheels. Then, push yourself away from the bed, and position yourself properly in the wheelchair.

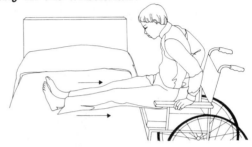

4 To get back into bed, position the wheelchair seat so it's facing the bed. Remove your legs from the legrests. Then, swing the legrests out of the way. Now, raise your legs onto the bed as you position the chair as close as possible to the bed. Lock the chair's wheels.

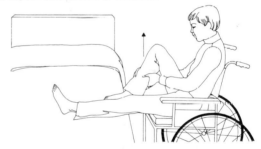

5 Next, grasp the armrests of the wheelchair, and lift your buttocks slightly off the seat. Keeping your legs extended across the bed, inch forward to the middle of the bed.

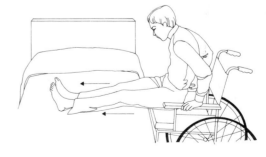

Performing transfers

How to use a patient roller board

1 *Consider this possibility: Jody Mayfield, a 26-year-old dietitian, is returning to the short-stay unit from the recovery room after a left inguinal herniorrhaphy. You decide to use a patient roller board to move him from the OR stretcher to a stretcher in the short-stay unit. To perform this transfer properly, follow these steps:*

First, enlist the help of a coworker. Then, explain the procedure to your patient. Loosen the bed linen on the OR stretcher, lower the side rails, and unfasten the safety straps on the stretcher.

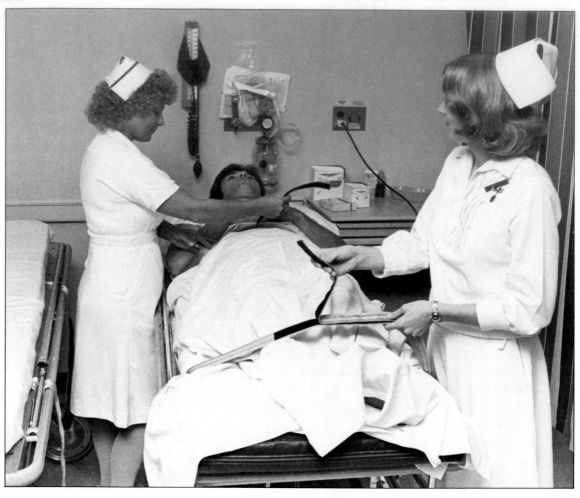

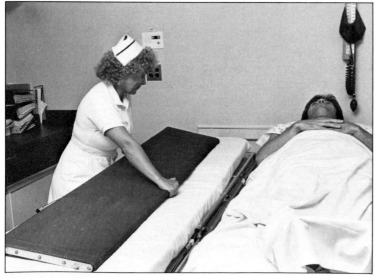

2 Lock the OR stretcher's wheels. Then, position the right side of the OR stretcher against the left side of the second stretcher, and lock the stretcher's wheels. Place the roller board on the second stretcher, as shown here.

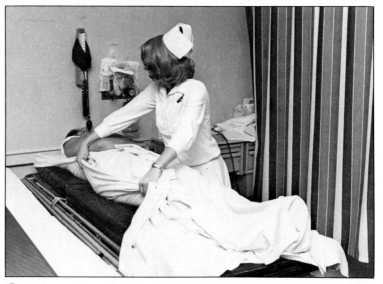

3 Tell your coworker to stand at the left side of the OR stretcher, facing you. Instruct her to reach over your patient and grasp the right side of the stretcher's sheet.

4 Next, ask your co-worker to lift the right side of the sheet slightly. As she does, slide the roller board under your patient. Make sure the board is under his right leg, hip, and shoulder. *Note:* You may have to kneel on the OR stretcher to slide the board under him.

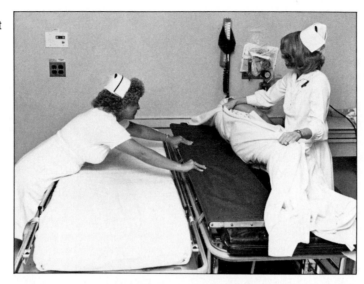

5 Instruct your co-worker to grasp the left side of the stretcher sheet, while you grasp the right side. On a predetermined signal, pull the right side of the sheet toward you, sliding your patient over the roller board. Your coworker will help guide him from the left side.

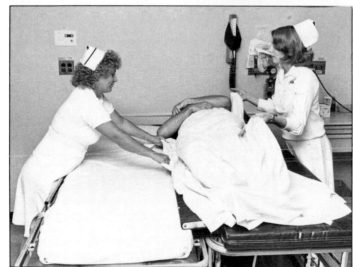

6 When your patient's on the second stretcher, raise the second stretcher's right side rail. Then, reach over your patient and grasp the left side of the sheet and lift your patient on his side. Instruct your co-worker to slide the roller board out from underneath your patient.

Position your patient properly, making sure his body's well aligned. Raise the left side rail. Document the procedure in your notes.

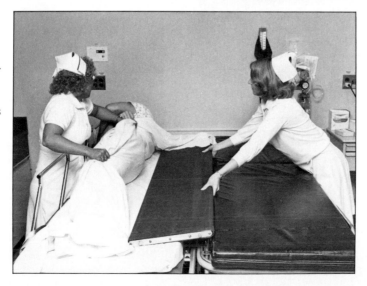

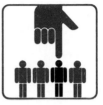

How to transfer a patient with halo traction
Does the thought of transferring a patient with halo traction make you uncomfortable? Don't let it. You can safely use a stand-pivot or a sitting transfer with a transfer board, as explained on pages 82 to 83 and 97. However, follow these precautions with either technique:
• Squat slightly to position your head below your patient's halo, as shown.
• You can place towels or foam padding between your patient's halo and your head. This will prevent you from accidentally hitting the halo with your head or upper body.
• *Caution:* Never grasp any part of your patient's halo.

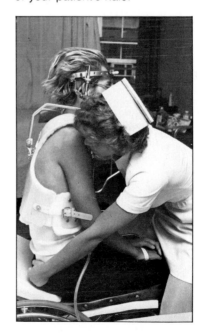

Performing transfers

Using a Trans-Aid® institutional lifter to move your patient from a bed to a wheelchair

1 *Let's say you want to transfer 38-year-old Richard Cantwell from his bed to a wheelchair. Mr. Cantwell suffers severe overall body weakness from a spinal tumor. Because he's too heavy for you to move by yourself—and you don't want to strain your back— you decide to use a mechanical lifter.*

In this photostory, we've used the Trans-Aid® institutional lifter and sling. If you're using another type of mechanical lifter, consult the manufacturer's instructions before you begin.

Place a wheelchair to the left of the bed, leaving enough room to operate the lifter. Lock the chair's wheels, and move the legrests out of the way.

Next, thoroughly explain the procedure to your patient and reassure him. If he might need mechanical lifting at home, take this opportunity to explain the procedure to his family, also.

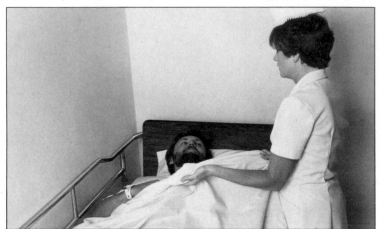

3 Roll your patient onto his left side, and unfold the sling. Place him in a supine position in the center of the sling, with his body well aligned.

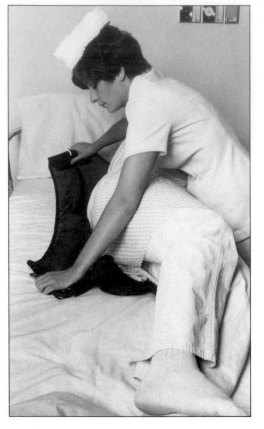

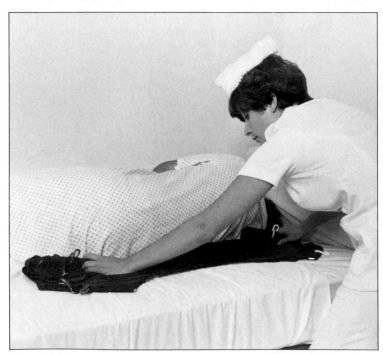

2 Roll Mr. Cantwell onto his right side. Fanfold the sling, and place it behind him. Position all hooks with the open ends away from his body. Make sure the white hooks are next to his right shoulder and the gold hooks are behind his right knee.

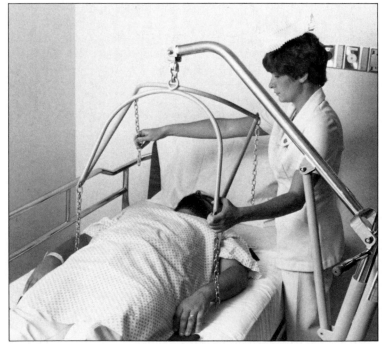

4 Now, position the Trans-Aid institutional lifter above your patient, as shown here.

Attach the white hooks to the silver chain and the gold hooks to the gold chain.

5 Firmly turn the handle of the lifter clockwise to raise Mr. Cantwell to a sitting position. Then, stop turning and check to be sure he's positioned properly. If he's not, lower him to the bed by turning the handle counter-clockwise, and re-position the sling. If everything's OK, continue to raise the sling until your patient's suspended just above the bed. Keep your arm under your patient's knees during the procedure, to guide him.

[Inset] Next, slowly turn the sling so your patient's legs hang over the edge of the bed.

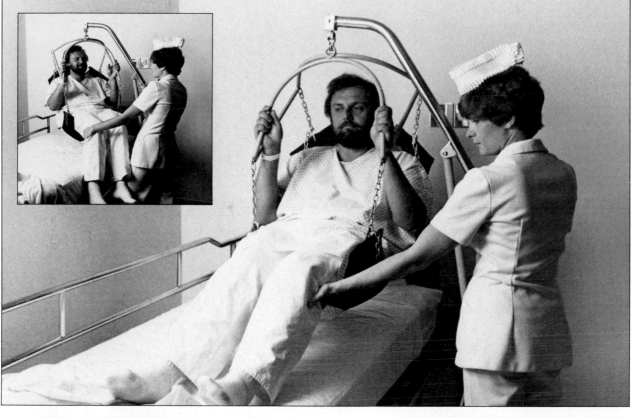

6 Carefully move the lifter toward the wheelchair, reassuring your patient as you do. Now, position him directly above the wheelchair's seat.

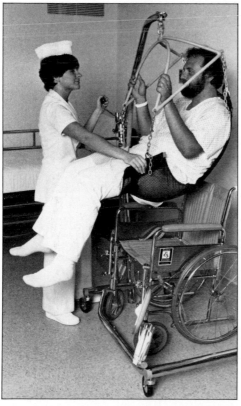

7 Slowly turn the lifter's handle counterclockwise to lower him onto the seat. When the chains become slack, stop turning.

Unhook the sling from the lifter. Leave the sling under your patient if he'll only be in the chair a short time, or you can remove it to make him more comfortable. To prevent skin irritation, smooth any folds you see in the sling material. Then, position your patient correctly in the chair. Document what you've done in your nurses' notes.

Remember: Reverse this entire procedure to move your patient back to bed from the wheelchair.

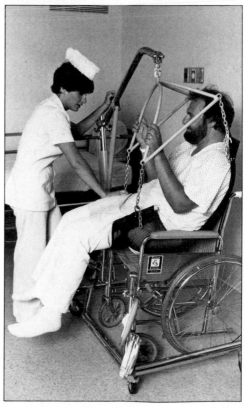

Performing transfers

Using a Trans-Aid® institutional lifter to transfer your patient into a car

1 *Let's assume Mr. Cantwell's been discharged and you want to move him into his car with a mechanical lifter. You'll follow these steps:*

Important: Before you begin, measure the width of the sling cradle and compare it with the car door opening. (In some cars, the door is too narrow to allow this type of transfer.)

Now, thoroughly review the procedure with your patient and reassure him. At this time, you may also want to reinforce what you taught his family about the lifter.

Then, make sure the car's parked close to the door of the building, on a level surface. Allow enough room for the lifter on the right side of the car.

Now, open the car's front door as far as possible, as shown here.

Position your patient in the Trans-Aid institutional lifter, with his hands inside the cradle.

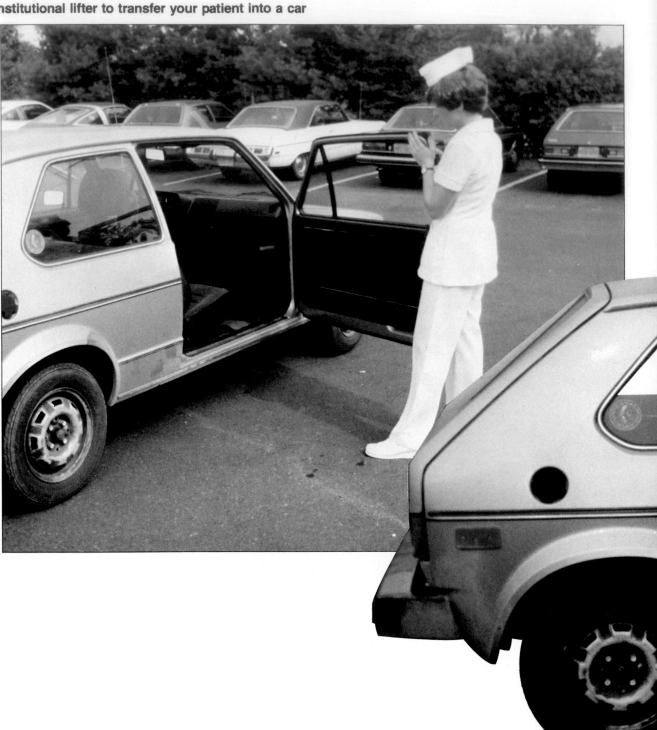

2 Slowly wheel the lifter over to the car. Position the lifter so your patient's directly in front of the door opening, as shown in this photo. Make sure the lifter's front wheels are under the car.

3 Now, turn the lifter's handle to lower the cross arm so it clears the car roof. Make sure your patient's head also clears the car roof.

Push the lifter so the cradle enters the car. Position your patient's buttocks over the car seat. When you complete this procedure, your patient will be sitting with his legs dangling outside the car.

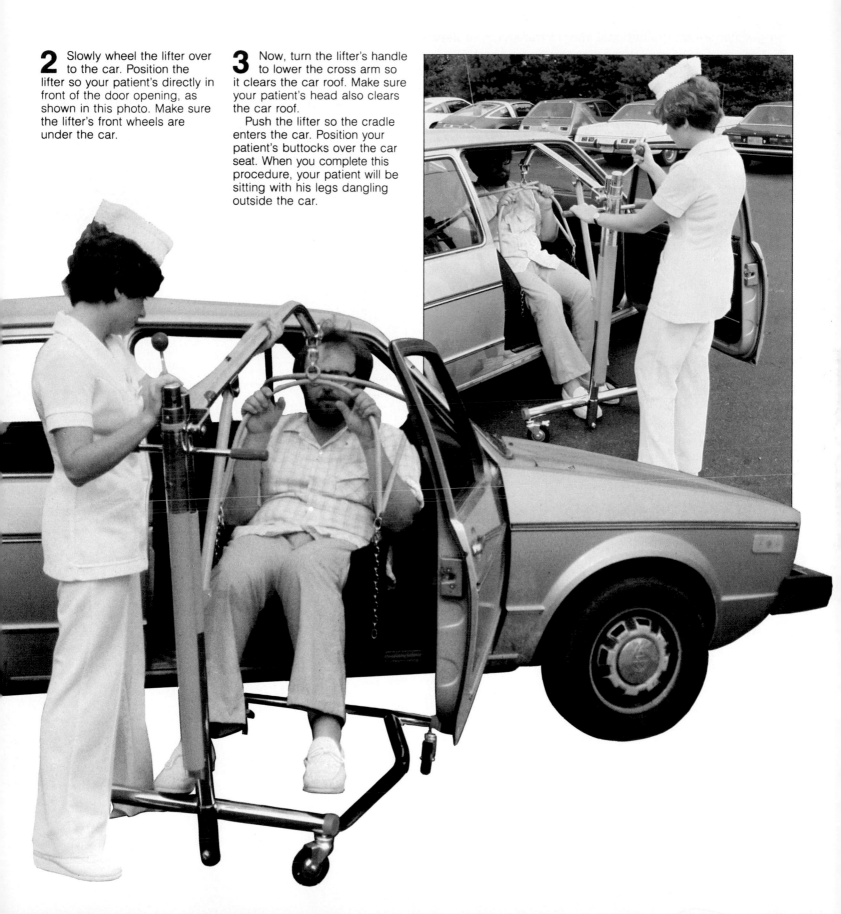

Performing transfers

Using a Trans-Aid® institutional lifter to transfer your patient into a car continued

4 Next, remove the chains from the hooks on the sling. Move the lifter out of the way. Tuck the left side of the sling behind your patient's back. Then, place your hands under his knees and lift his legs into the car, as the nurse is doing here. Ask your patient to guide himself with his arms, if he can.

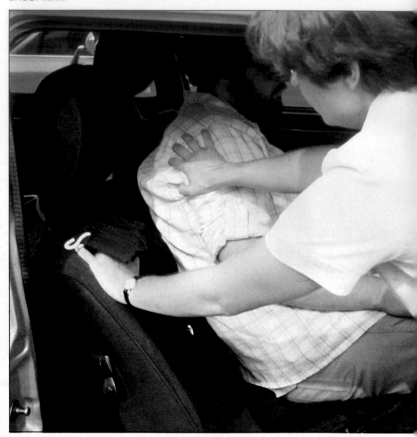

5 Now, lean your patient toward his left side. Tell him to hold onto the dashboard as you slowly pull the sling out from under him.

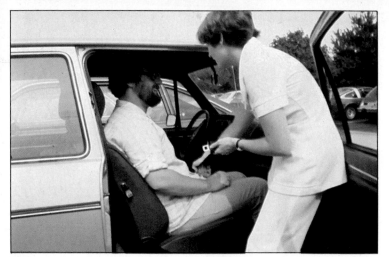

6 Then, make sure your patient's properly positioned in the seat. His feet should be flat on the floor. Adjust the car seat, if necessary. Finally, secure your patient's seat belt, and shut the car door.

Using a transfer board: Some suggestions

As you know, a sitting transfer with a transfer board is a simple method to use for transferring a patient. But, before you use a transfer board, always check your patient's buttocks for signs of skin breakdown. If your patient's a male, also check his scrotal area for irritation.

Suppose you see a reddened or blanched area on your patient's skin. Choose another transfer method immediately. The transfer board will further irritate his skin.

 Nursing tip: As an additional precaution against skin irritation, make sure your patient's wearing pajama bottoms, or cover the transfer board with a disposable underpad or drawsheet. By doing this, you'll reduce friction between the board and your patient's skin.

Sitting transfer: Teaching your patient how to use a transfer board

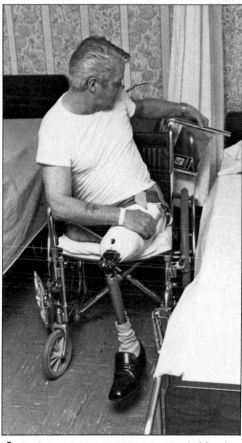

1 *Let's assume you want to teach Marvin Goldberg, a 63-year-old pharmacist, how to transfer himself from his wheelchair to his bed. Do you know how? If you're unsure, follow these steps:*

First, explain the procedure to your patient, and assure him you'll help, if necessary. Then, make sure his wheelchair has removable armrests and legrests. Ask him to move his wheelchair next to the bed, so the left side of the chair is next to the right side of the bed. Have him lock the chair's wheels in place.

Remove the wheelchair's legrests for Mr. Goldberg. Also, adjust his bed so it's level with the wheelchair seat.

Now, he'll remove the wheelchair's left armrest and hang it from the back of the chair, as shown here.

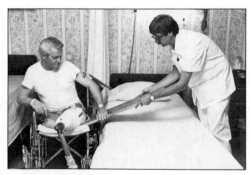

2 Have Mr. Goldberg shift his weight onto his right buttock. Now, help him slide the transfer board under his buttocks and upper thighs. Instruct him to extend the other end of the board onto the bed.

Tell Mr. Goldberg to make sure the board is resting securely on the wheelchair seat and the bed.

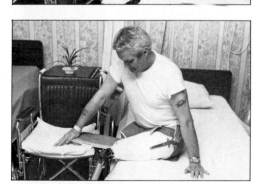

3 Next, have your patient grasp the chair's right armrest with his right hand, and place his left hand on the transfer board. Then, he'll lift his buttocks and begin to inch his way across the board, toward the bed, as shown in this photo.

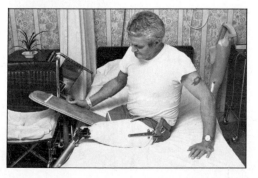

4 When Mr. Goldberg reaches the bed, have him place his left hand on the bed. His right hand will be on the transfer board.

5 Next, as he grasps the transfer board with his right hand, tell him to shift his weight to his left hip. Then, have him pull the board from underneath himself. Have him replace the armrest and legrests.

Performing transfers

Sitting transfer: How to move a patient using a transfer board

1 *What if you're caring for Steve Stabile, a 23-year-old mechanic with newly diagnosed multiple sclerosis? Mr. Stabile can't independently transfer himself with a transfer board. So, you'll have to assist him with the transfer. Here's how:*

Before you begin, explain the procedure. Then, make sure you have the following: a transfer belt, a wheelchair with removable armrests, and a transfer board.

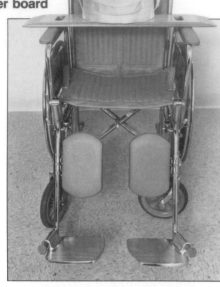

2 Now, move the wheelchair next to the bed. Make sure the right side of the chair is next to the left side of the bed. Lock the chair's wheels and the bed wheels in place. Remove the wheelchair's right armrest and both legrests, if possible.

Note: If the legrests aren't removable, raise the foot pedals, and position the legrests as close to the bed as possible.

Adjust your patient's bed so it's level with the wheelchair seat.

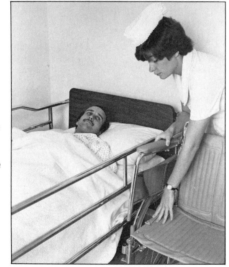

3 Now help your patient dangle his legs over the side of the bed. Put shoes on his feet, and secure a transfer belt around his waist.

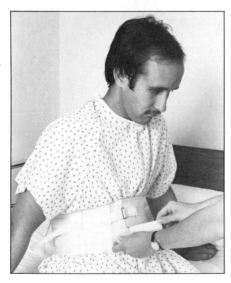

4 Next, have your patient shift his weight onto his right buttock, and carefully slide the transfer board under him. Place the other end of the board on the wheelchair seat, making sure it's secure on both ends.

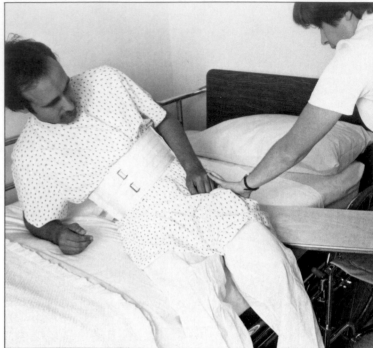

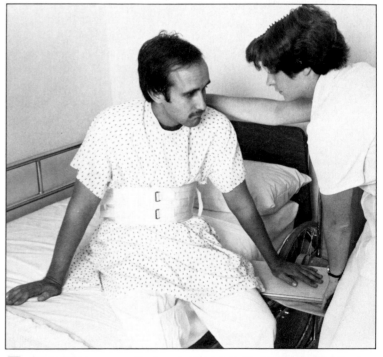

5 Reposition your patient upright and angle his body slightly, as he's sitting on the transfer board.

Stand facing your patient. Place your legs on either side of his legs.

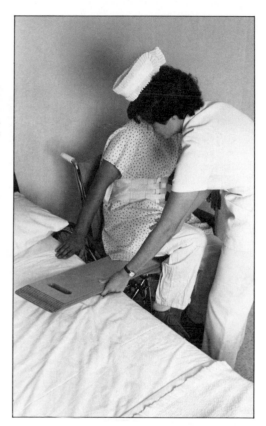

7 Carefully, with one continuous motion, guide your patient across the transfer board toward the wheelchair. If necessary, you can stop to rest or reposition your patient before completing the transfer.

When he's close to the seat of the wheelchair, lean his body toward the left side of the chair.

Gently raise his right leg and ease the transfer board out from under him.

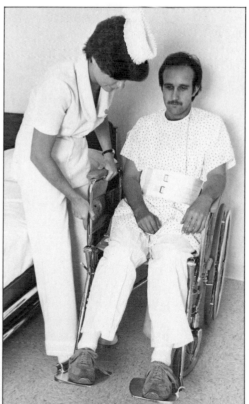

8 Position him properly in the wheelchair. Replace the chair's armrest and legrests.

Document the procedure in your nurses' notes and the patient's positioning schedule.

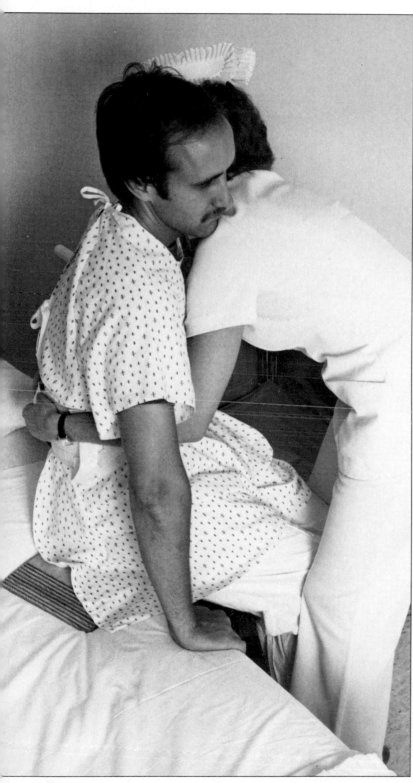

6 Next, squat down so his chin is resting on your left shoulder. Instruct him to press his chin against your shoulder for balance. Wrap your arms around his upper body, and grasp the back of his transfer belt.

Performing transfers

How to perform a car transfer with a transfer board

1 *Imagine this situation: Steve Stabile is being discharged. Mr. Stabile's been using a transfer board to move from his bed to a wheelchair and will continue to use the board at home. Do you know how to help him use a transfer board to move from his wheelchair into a car? Follow these steps:*

First, explain the transfer technique you'll be using to Mr. Stabile, and ask him to help as much as possible. Place a transfer belt around his waist, and make sure his wheelchair has a removable armrest. Open the car's front passenger door as far as possible. Then, carefully push the wheelchair, and Mr. Stabile, over to the door.

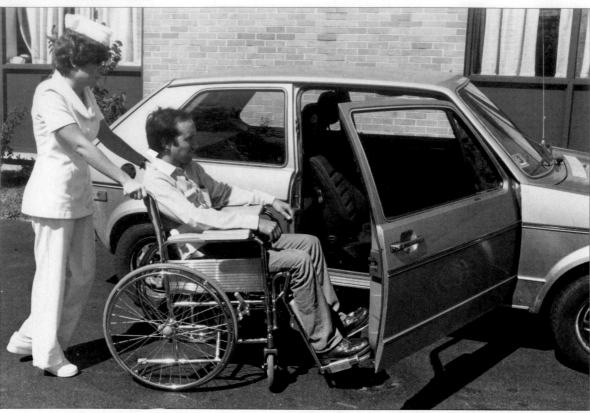

2 Now, lock the wheels of the chair. Remove the left armrest and both legrests, if possible.

Position the wheelchair's seat so it's parallel to the car seat. Mr. Stabile should face the *front* of the car.

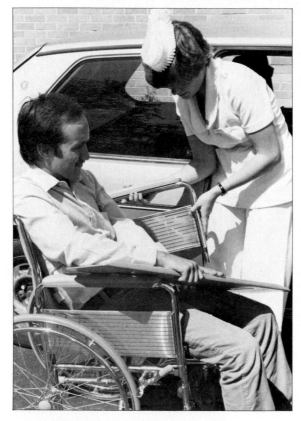

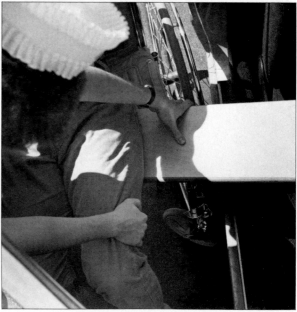

3 Ask Mr. Stabile to shift his weight to his right buttock. Then, position the end of the transfer board under his left buttock. Slide the board under his right buttock and upper right thigh. Then, make sure he's sitting with both buttocks on the board.

Extend the other end of the board onto the car seat, making sure it's secure.

4 Instruct Mr. Stabile to place his hands on the board. Tell him to lift his buttocks slightly off the board by pushing downward with his hands. Then, tell him to inch his way across the board toward the car seat.

[Inset] What if Mr. Stabile is too weak to inch himself along the board? Then, grasp his transfer belt, and guide him along the board toward the car seat.

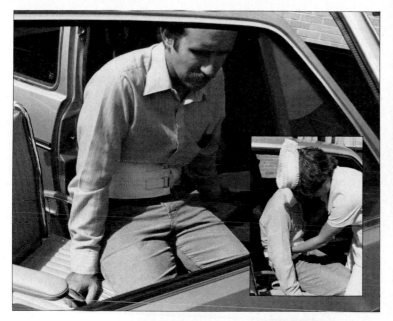

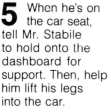

5 When he's on the car seat, tell Mr. Stabile to hold onto the dashboard for support. Then, help him lift his legs into the car.

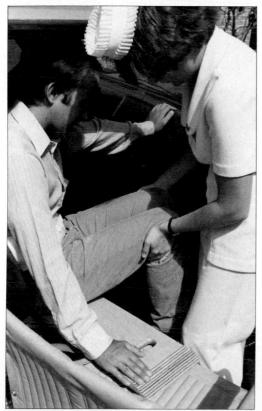

6 To remove the board, he'll grasp the transfer board with his right hand, and shift his weight to his left hip. Tell him to pull the board from underneath himself, or remove the board for him, as the nurse is doing here. If the board belongs to him, have him put it in the car.

Suppose Mr. Stabile's left side is weakened. Reverse the transfer direction explained here, and transfer him—right side first—onto the back seat, directly behind the driver. However, don't try this unless the car has four doors. Never transfer a patient into the driver's side of a car, because the steering wheel will get in the way.

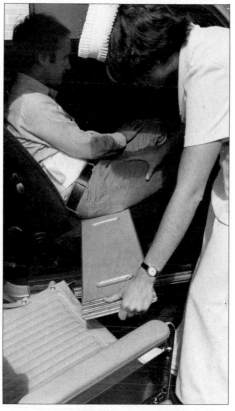

7 Replace the wheelchair's armrest and legrests. Then, if the chair belongs to the patient, fold it and place it in the back seat or trunk. If the chair doesn't belong to him, make sure the family has made arrangements to secure one.

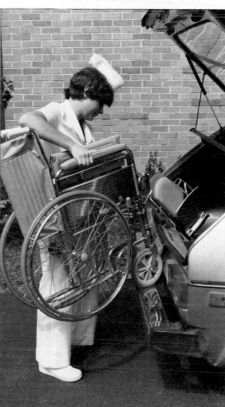

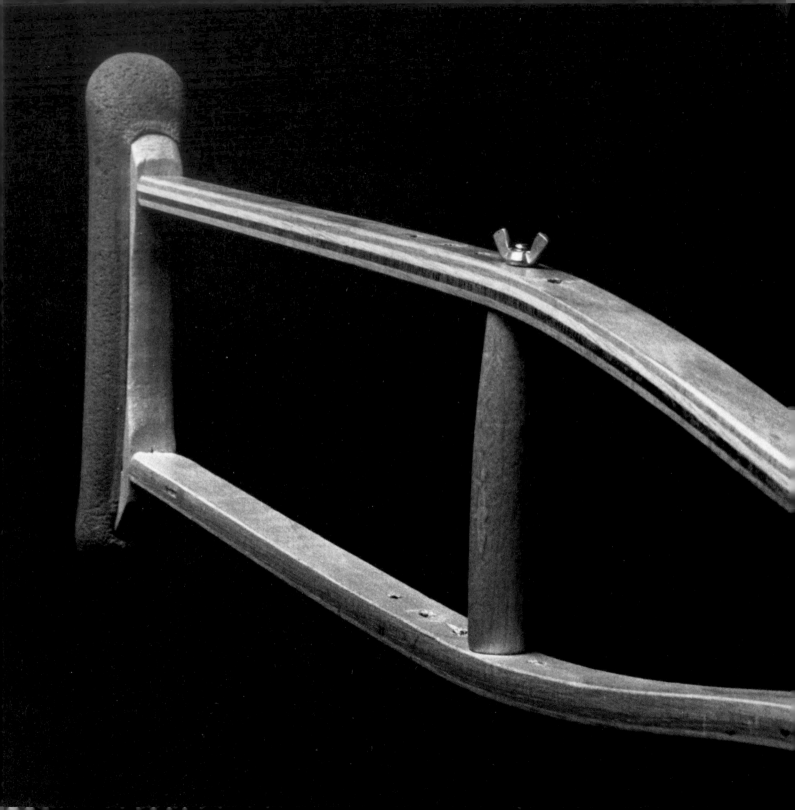

Aiding Mobility with Special Equipment

Crutches, canes, and walkers

Wheelchairs

Crutches, canes, and walkers

Are you recommending or selecting crutches, a cane, or a walker for your patient? If so, how familiar are you with various sizes and types of these mobility aids? Do you know when your patient needs a half-circle cane or a reciprocal walker? Can you determine if your patient's crutches are the correct size?

On the following pages, we'll show you:
- how to teach your patient to walk with two canes.
- how to teach your patient to climb a flight of stairs using crutches or a cane.
- how to teach your patient to get in and out of a chair with crutches, a cane, or a walker.

The step-by-step photos and illustrations will help you assist your patient with the following gaits: two-point, three-point, three-point-and-one, swing-through three-point, and four-point. We've also included numerous nursing tips to make your job easier. Read this part of the book carefully.

Do your patient's crutches fit properly?

You know how important it is for your patient to use properly fitting crutches. But do you know how to evaluate the size and safety of his crutches? Whenever a doctor or physical therapist orders crutches for your patient, check the crutches thoroughly. Avoid possible accidents by following these guidelines:
- *Check safety features.* Make sure the crutches have rubber tips to prevent slipping, and rubber pads at the top. Ask your patient if he wants the hand supports padded.
- *Check crutch size.* To do this, ask your patient to stand and position the crutch tips 2" (5 cm) in front of and 6" (15 cm) to the side of his feet. Make sure the tops of the crutches are about 1" to 1½" (two finger widths or 2.5 to 3.8 cm) below his axillae. If they're too long or too short, adjust them. Then recheck them.

Check the hand supports to make sure they're positioned correctly. To do this, ask your patient to grasp the supports with his arms slightly flexed, not straight. Also, ask him if he would like the hand supports padded. In addition, remind your patient to support his weight on his hands, not his axillae. Tell him that tingling or numbness in his upper torso may mean he's using the crutches incorrectly. Or, that the crutches are the wrong size.

Crutches, canes, and walkers: Some helpful hints

Planning to help your patient walk with crutches, a cane, or a walker? If so, here are some suggestions to remember:
- When possible, instruct your patient how to use his crutches, cane, or walker *before* he needs them; for example, before surgery.
- For added support, place a transfer or walking belt around your patient's waist before he begins.
- Make sure he's wearing well-fitting flat shoes.
- To avoid accidents, have your patient stand for several minutes with his crutches, cane, or walker, until he can maintain his balance. Remind him that some temporary dizziness is normal. However, if he seems excessively dizzy, lower him onto a bed or chair, and notify the doctor.
- Instruct your patient to look ahead when walking, instead of at his feet.
- Make sure the surface your patient will be walking on is clean, flat, dry, and well lighted.
- To prevent falls, stay with your patient as he's learning the procedure, and guide him through each gait. Stand behind and slightly to one side of him. (If he has unilateral weakness, stand close to the affected side.) Have one hand near his shoulder and the other prepared to grasp his transfer belt. By doing this, you can support him if he loses his balance.

Guidelines for gait selection

Preparing to assist your patient with crutch-walking? If so, you'll need to know which gait his doctor or physical therapist has chosen for him. Or, you may have to choose your patient's gait, after consulting the doctor (depending on hospital policy). To learn which gait is right for your patient, review the guidelines listed below:

Four-point gait

Choose a four-point gait if your patient can't support his full weight on either of his legs; for example, a patient with leg muscle weakness or spasticity, poor muscular coordination or balance, degenerative leg joint disease, or bilateral leg prostheses.

Two-point gait

Choose a two-point gait if your patient can't support his full weight on his legs but does have reasonably good muscular coordination and arm strength.

Three-point-and-one-gait (partial-weight–bearing)

Choose a three-point-and-one gait if your patient can support his full weight on one leg and partial weight on his other leg; for example, a patient with a walking cast, degenerative joint disease, or a new leg prosthesis. This gait may also be used by a patient who has had leg surgery.

Three-point gait (non-weight–bearing)

Choose a three-point gait if your patient can't support his weight on one leg but has normal use of his arms, upper body, and other leg; for example, a patient who's had one leg amputated but has no prosthesis, or a patient with musculoskeletal or soft-tissue trauma. Also, consider this gait for a patient who has an acute leg inflammation or has recently had leg surgery.

Swing-through three-point gait

Choose a swing-through three-point gait if your patient can't support weight on one leg but has good muscular strength and coordination; for example, a patient with spina bifida, paraplegia, or myelomeningocele. This gait allows the patient to ambulate faster than the other gaits and can be used with leg braces.

Crutch-walking: How to help your patient with the two-point gait

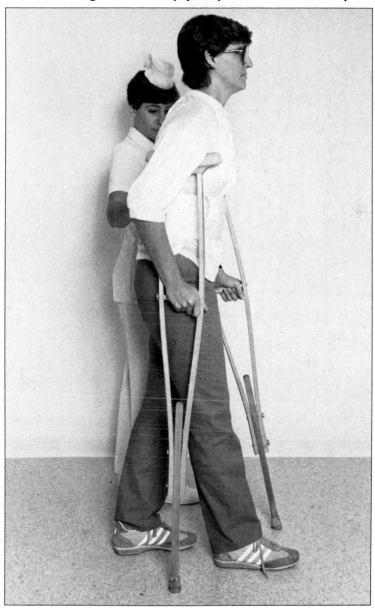

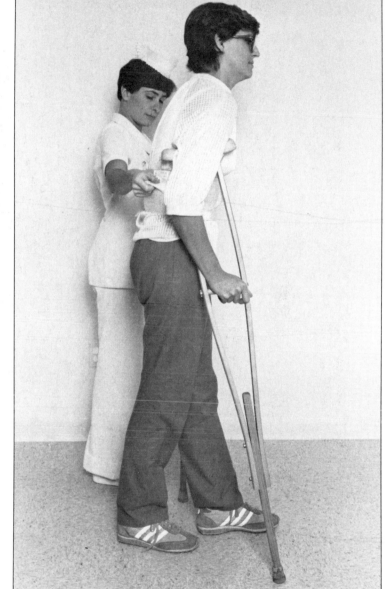

1 *Preparing to help your patient with the two-point gait? If so, proceed as follows:*
Begin by explaining the procedure to your patient. Place a transfer belt around her waist. Then, ask your patient to stand with her weight evenly distributed between both legs and crutches.

Stand behind her and slightly to the side. Tell your patient to shift her weight to her right crutch and left foot as she moves her left crutch and right foot about 8″ (20 cm) forward.

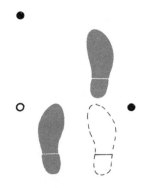

2 Now, instruct her to shift her weight to her left crutch and right foot as she moves her right crutch and her left foot approximately 8″ (20 cm) forward.

Have her repeat these steps. Stay with her until you're both confident she's mastered the gait.

Important: Use the diagrams at the bottom of these captions to visualize how the patient would be positioned if you were helping her.

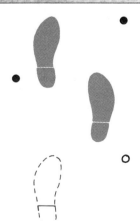

Crutches, canes, and walkers

Crutch-walking: How to help your patient with the four-point gait

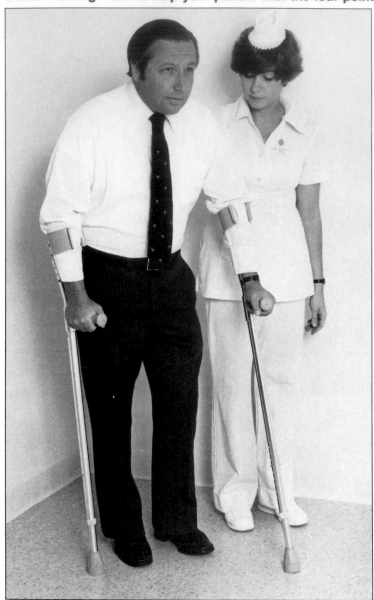

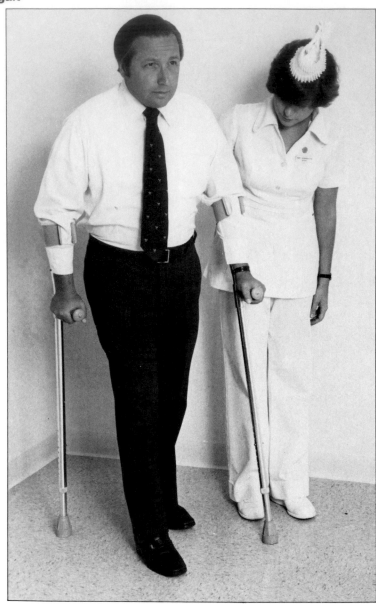

1 *Let's assume the doctor has instructed you to teach 40-year-old Antonio Bardoutsous the four-point gait. Mr. Bardoutsous lacks muscle coordination in his legs. Do you know how to proceed with the teaching session? If not, follow these guidelines:*

Explain the procedure. Support Mr. Bardoutsous by holding his belt. Tell him to stand with his weight evenly distributed between both legs and the crutches. Stand behind him and slightly to his side.

Now, tell Mr. Bardoutsous to move his left crutch about 8" (20 cm) forward. As he does, have him shift his weight so it's distributed evenly between his right crutch and both legs.

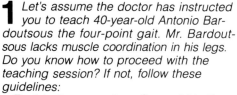

2 Next, tell your patient to move his right foot approximately 8" (20 cm) forward, so it's even with the left crutch.

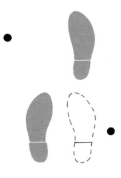

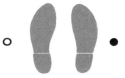

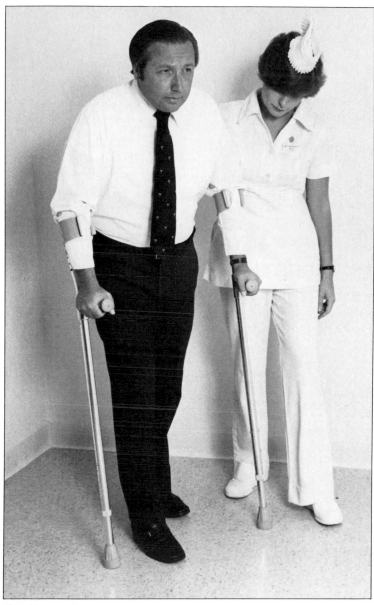

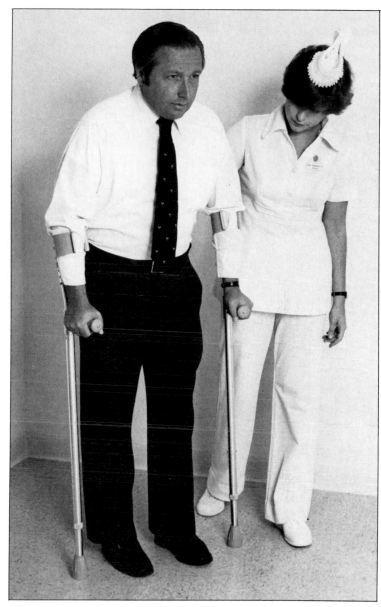

3 Now, ask your patient to move his right crutch about 8″ (20 cm) forward, as he shifts his weight onto his left crutch and both legs.

4 Tell him to move his left foot 8″ (20 cm) forward, even with his right crutch.
   Have him repeat this procedure—moving each crutch forward, then moving the opposite foot. Continue to reassure and encourage Mr. Bardoutsous until you're both confident he's mastered the gait.

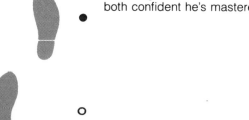

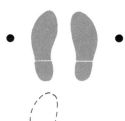

Crutches, canes, and walkers

How to teach your patient the three-point gait (non-weight–bearing)

1 *You're ready to teach 23-year-old Jane Hippler how to crutch-walk using a three-point gait. Jane's left ankle is sprained and wrapped with an elastic bandage. Do you know how to proceed? Follow these steps carefully:*

First, explain the procedure. Then, standing at the side of the chair, help her slide to the edge. Her right foot should be flat on the floor. Make sure she's wearing a shoe on her right foot. Instruct her to hold both crutches in her left hand, as shown here.

Direct Jane to lean forward from her waist, advancing her right foot slightly ahead of her left foot. Tell her to place her right hand on the arm of the chair. As she steadies herself with the crutches, tell her to push herself up with her hand and support all her weight with her right leg.

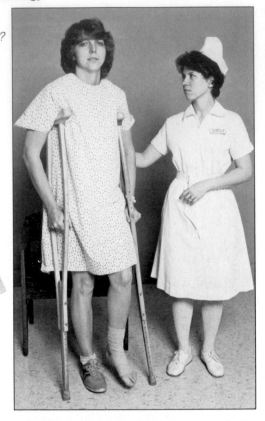

2 When she's standing, instruct Jane to transfer one crutch to her right side and grasp it firmly. Encourage her to relax her shoulders. Remind her to keep her left foot off the floor as she flexes her left knee slightly. Have her position her right foot so it's even with the crutch tips.

Use the diagrams at the bottom of these captions to visualize how the patient will be positioned if *you* were helping her.

3 When Jane can maintain her balance, instruct her to lean her body slightly forward. Have her support her weight on her right foot and the crutches.

Position yourself behind her, slightly to her left side.

Now, tell her to shift her weight to her right leg and move both crutches forward. Then, she'll swing her left leg forward. Remind her not to put weight on her left foot.

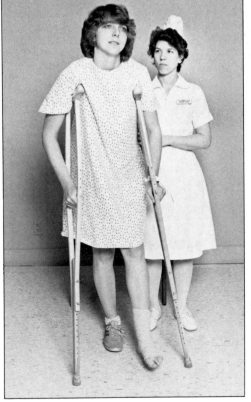

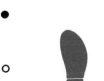

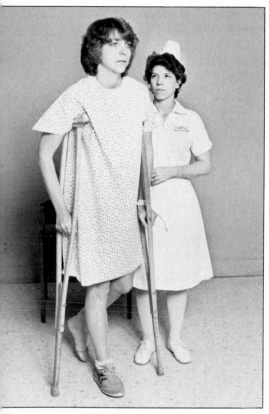

4 Next, have Jane balance her weight on both crutches as she swings her right leg forward, as shown here.

Ask Jane to put her weight on her right leg, using her crutches to maintain her balance.

Then, have her move both crutches and her left foot forward and repeat the procedure.

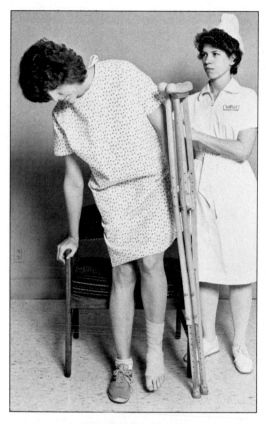

6 When she's ready to return to her chair, instruct her to move her left leg as close as possible to the chair. Ask Jane to transfer both crutches to her left hand as she places her right hand on the armrest, as shown in this photo.

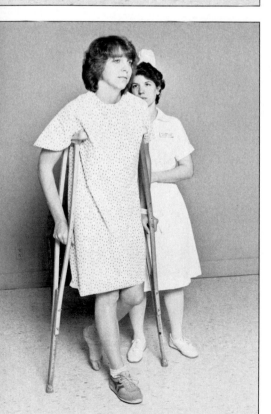

5 As your patient's balance and strength improve, teach her the swing-through three-point gait. To do this, instruct Jane to advance her right foot beyond the crutches. Then she'll advance both crutches and her left leg past her right foot, as shown. Have her repeat the procedure.

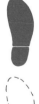

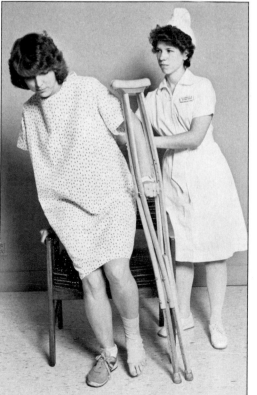

7 Tell her to slowly pivot until the backs of her knees touch the chair seat. As she supports her weight on her hand and the crutches, instruct her to slowly lower herself onto the seat.

Remind Jane to keep her crutches within easy reach.

Crutches, canes, and walkers

Crutch-walking: How to teach your patient the three-point-and-one gait (partial-weight–bearing)

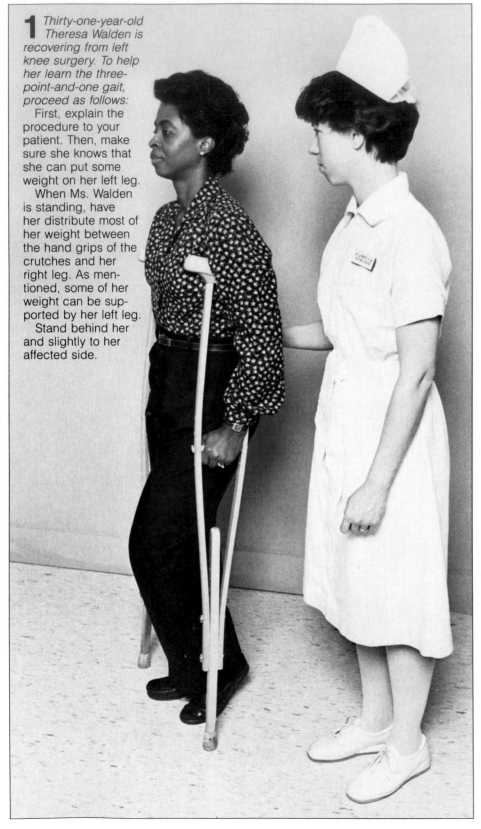

1 *Thirty-one-year-old Theresa Walden is recovering from left knee surgery. To help her learn the three-point-and-one gait, proceed as follows:*
    First, explain the procedure to your patient. Then, make sure she knows that she can put some weight on her left leg.
    When Ms. Walden is standing, have her distribute most of her weight between the hand grips of the crutches and her right leg. As mentioned, some of her weight can be supported by her left leg.
    Stand behind her and slightly to her affected side.

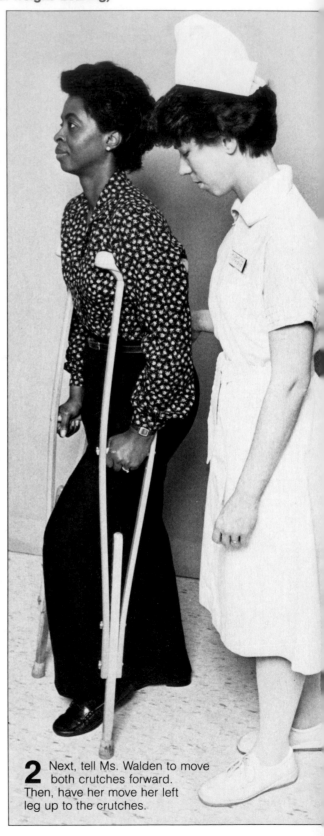

2 Next, tell Ms. Walden to move both crutches forward. Then, have her move her left leg up to the crutches.

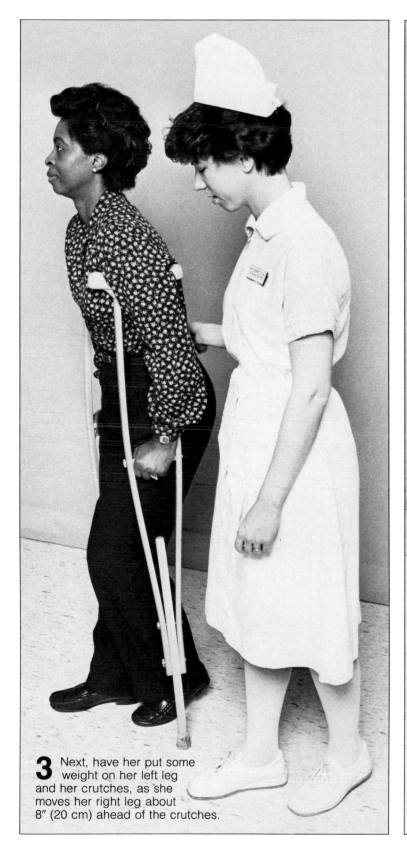

3 Next, have her put some weight on her left leg and her crutches, as she moves her right leg about 8″ (20 cm) ahead of the crutches.

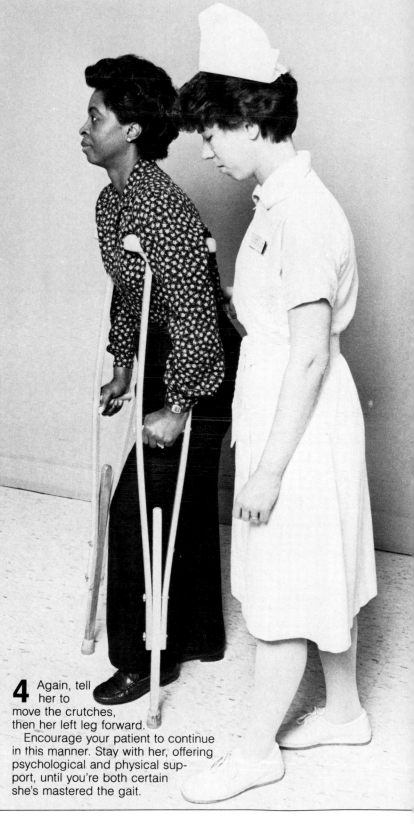

4 Again, tell her to move the crutches, then her left leg forward.
   Encourage your patient to continue in this manner. Stay with her, offering psychological and physical support, until you're both certain she's mastered the gait.

Crutches, canes, and walkers

How to help a patient with crutches in and out of a chair

1 *You're caring for 9-year-old Andy Sero, who sprained his left ankle playing baseball. Andy has just learned to walk with crutches. Here's how to teach him to get in and out of a chair.*

Begin by explaining the procedure to your patient. Then have him approach the chair so his right leg's close to the chair seat. Tell him to grasp both crutches with his left hand.

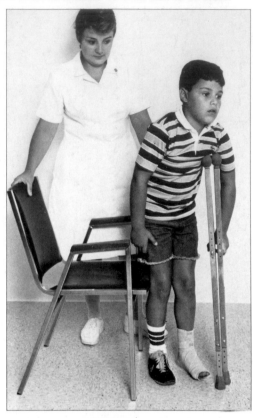

2 Next, tell Andy to put his right hand on the arm of the chair. Have him place the crutches at the back of the chair, as shown here.

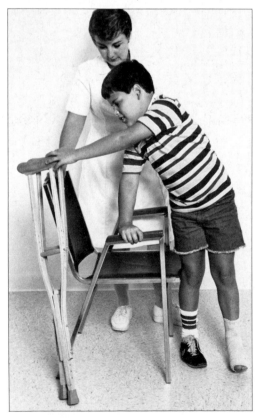

3 Now, instruct your patient to pivot on his right foot until the back of his right leg is against the seat of the chair. Ask him to place his left hand on the arm of the chair.

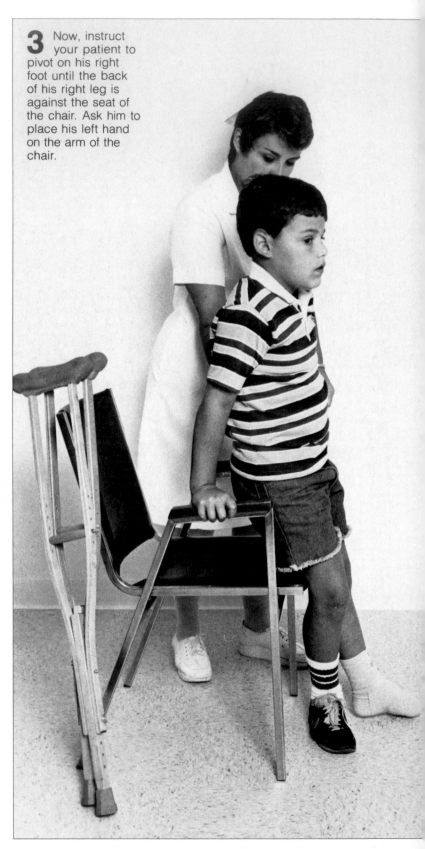

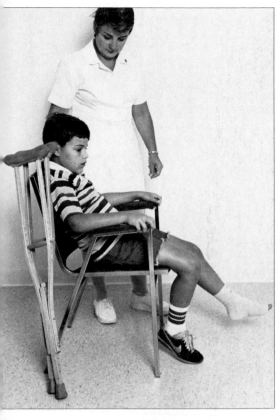

4 As he supports his weight with his hands, have him lower himself into the chair.

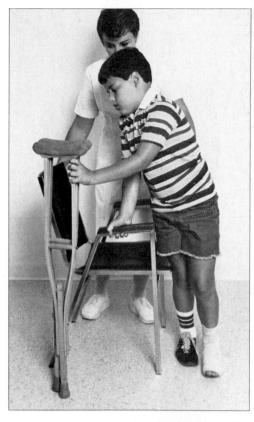

6 Next, ask your patient to pivot on his right foot, while grasping the armrest with his right hand. He'll grasp the crutches with his left hand.

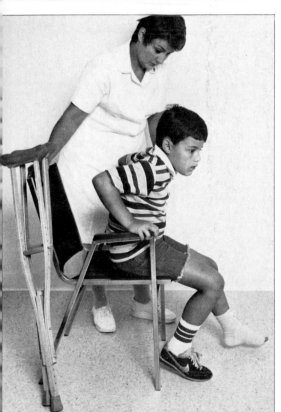

5 Now, let's suppose he wants to get out of the chair. Tell Andy to slide forward, keeping his right foot slightly under the chair. Have him press down on the armrests, as shown here.

Now, instruct Andy to support his weight on his hands and right foot as he lifts himself out of the chair.

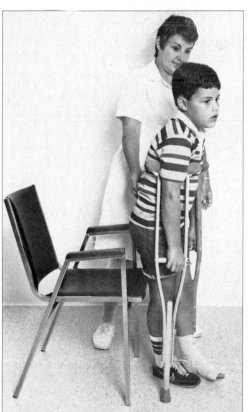

7 Finally, tell him to place both crutches under his left arm. As soon as he feels steady, tell him to shift one crutch to his right arm. Andy is now ready to walk.

Document the teaching session in your nurses' notes.

Crutches, canes, and walkers

Crutch-walking: How to help your patient go up and down stairs

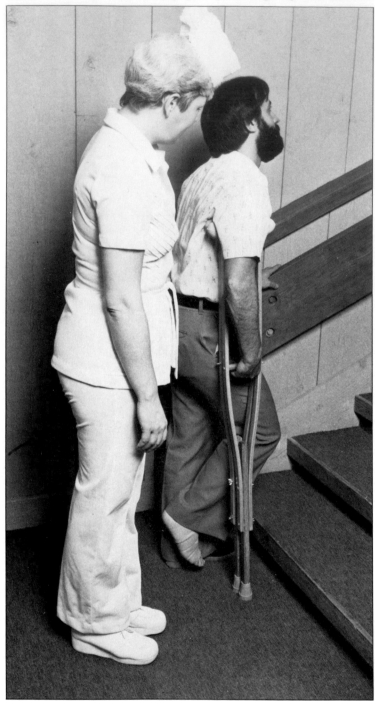

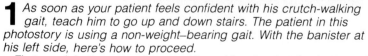

1 As soon as your patient feels confident with his crutch-walking gait, teach him to go up and down stairs. The patient in this photostory is using a non-weight–bearing gait. With the banister at his left side, here's how to proceed.

First, explain the procedure, and have him stand at the bottom of the stairs. Stand behind him, slightly to his right.

Instruct your patient to grasp the banister with his left hand and shift his left crutch to his right hand. Have him support his weight on both crutches and his left leg.

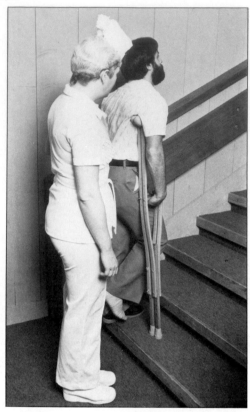

2 Tell your patient to push down on his crutches and hop onto the first step with his left foot. His other leg will move up onto the step at the same time.

Next, have your patient swing his crutches up onto the first step, alongside his feet.

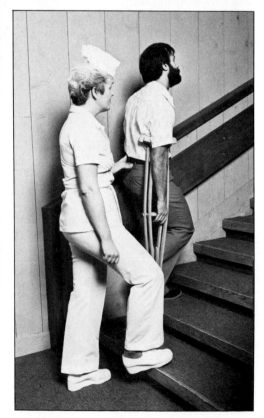

3 Ask him to hop onto the second step with his left leg.

Encourage your patient to repeat this procedure, advancing his left leg first, until he reaches the top of the stairs.

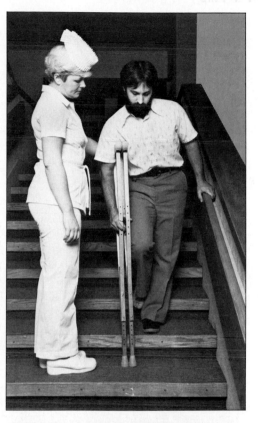

5 As you continue to support and encourage your patient, ask him to lower his crutches to the next step.

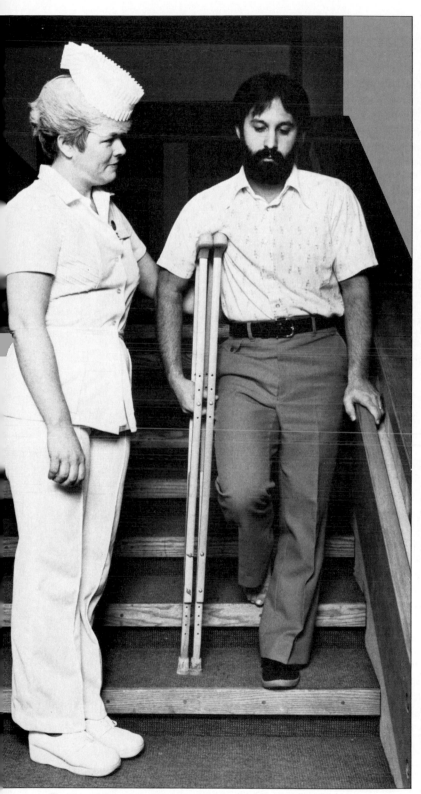

4 Now, show him how to get down the stairs. To do this, instruct him to grasp the banister and shift his left crutch to his right hand. Stand one step below.

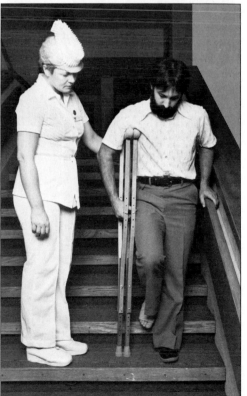

6 Next, tell him to lower his left foot onto the first step. As he does, his other leg will follow.

Have him repeat this procedure, advancing the crutches and his left leg first.

Important: If your patient is using the three-point-and-one gait, he'll simultaneously lower his right leg and both crutches.

Crutches, canes, and walkers

Choosing the proper cane for your patient

Canes come in a variety of sizes and styles. So, if you're helping select a cane for your patient, you'll want to know which size and style best suits his needs. Ask yourself these questions:
• *Will my patient's diagnosis or prognosis require a particular type of cane?* For example, if he has poor balance, he'll probably need a broad-based cane.
• *How tall is my patient?* Select the correct size cane, or choose a cane that's adjustable. To determine if your patient's cane is the proper size, ask him to stand with the cane's tip 4″ (10 cm) to the side of his foot. The cane should extend from the floor to his hip joint. As he holds it, his elbow should be flexed at a 30° angle.
• *Does the cane you're considering have a rubber tip?* A rubber tip keeps the cane from slipping and helps prevent accidents.
   Now, study the following pages to learn even more about canes.

Lumex Ortho-Ease Quad Cane (broad-based)

Description
• A metal cane with three or four prongs or legs to provide a wide base of support
• Bases range from narrow (4½″ x 7½″ [11.5 to 19cm]) to wide (12″ x 13½″ [30.5 to 34 cm]).
• Height can be adjusted from 30″ to 39″ (76 to 99 cm).
• Extra-long handles and child sizes are also available.
• A broad-based cane stands upright when released.

Nursing considerations
• Recommend a broad-based cane for a patient with poor balance.
• Encourage your patient to keep his body erect as he walks and not to lean out over the cane.
• Recommend your patient use a cane with as small a base as possible, and eventually progress to a single-ended cane, if he can. Remember, the smaller the base, the less the patient tends to rely on the cane for support.
• If your patient's using a broad-based cane, remind him to walk as close to the wall as possible. This will prevent others from kicking or tripping over the cane.
• A narrow broad-based cane fits on the standard stair step in the normal cane position. If your patient's using a wide broad-based cane, have him turn the cane sideways to fit on the step.

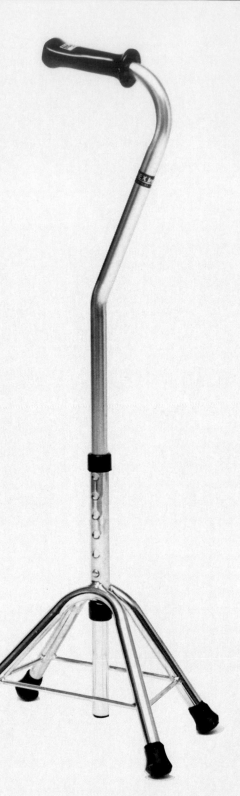

Lumex Ortho-Ease straight-handled cane

Description

• Wooden, plastic, or metal single-ended canes, with straight handles
• T-handle available in 34″ to 36″ sizes (86 to 91 cm). The J-line's available in 34″ to 44″ (86 to 112 cm) sizes. Some T-handle and J-line canes are adjustable.

Nursing considerations

• Recommend the T-handle or J-line cane for a patient with hand weakness. These canes have straight handles, with hand grips, which are easier to hold.
• Discourage use of this type of cane if your patient has poor balance.
• Make sure the handle of your patient's cane is the proper thickness for his hand.
• Remind your patient to place his T-handle or J-line cane on the floor when he's not using it. These canes can't be hooked over a chair arm or back, or leaned against a chair or bed.
• Encourage your patient to keep his body erect as he walks and not to lean out over the cane.

Regular cane

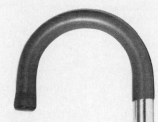

Description

• A wooden or metal single-ended cane, with a half-circle handle; usually inexpensive and easy to use
• Usually available in 34″ to 42″ (86 to 106 cm) sizes

Nursing considerations

• If the patient's doctor or physical therapist says he can use a cane, recommend a regular cane if he'll be going up and down stairs often. Instruct him to hook the cane to his belt or arm when he's going up and down stairs.
• Instruct your patient to hook a regular cane over a chair arm or back when he sits down, so it'll be within reach.
• Suggest your patient use a cane with a wooden or plastic handle rather than a metal one. If his hand perspires, he may lose his grip on a metal handle. Also, a metal handle may be uncomfortable in cold weather.
• Encourage your patient to keep his body erect as he walks and not to lean out over the cane.

Crutches, canes, and walkers

How to walk with a cane

1 *Your patient, 65-year-old Martha Samuels, is experiencing left-sided weakness from Parkinson's disease. The doctor asks you to help Mrs. Samuels with her cane-walking. Do you know how to proceed? Follow these steps:*

Note: In this photostory, Mrs. Samuels is using a Guardian Quadripoise® cane.

Begin by explaining the procedure to Mrs. Samuels, and reassure her. Make sure she's wearing nonskid shoes and check that her cane is the right height.

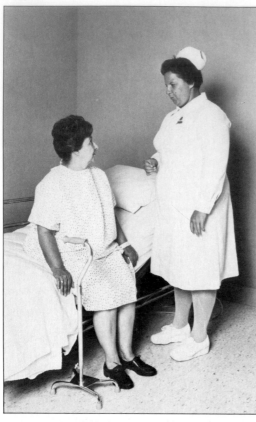

2 Now tell Mrs. Samuels to slide to the edge of the bed and place her feet flat on the floor 6" (15.2 cm) apart. Help her into a standing position. Stand slightly to Mrs. Samuels' weakened side.

Have her hold the cane in her right hand, with the tip about 4" (10.2 cm) to the side of her right foot. Tell her to distribute her weight evenly between her feet and the cane. Also remind her to keep the cane's rubber tips on the floor at all times.

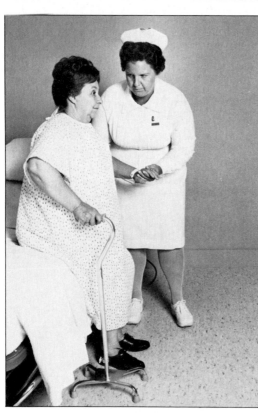

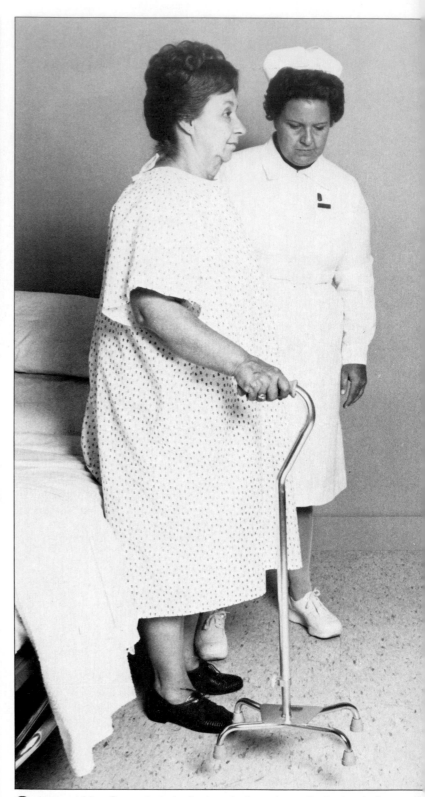

3 Instruct Mrs. Samuels to look ahead when she walks instead of looking at her feet. Then, ask your patient to shift her weight to her right leg as she moves the cane forward about 4" (10.2 cm).

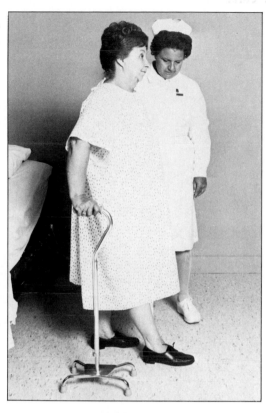

5 Now, with her weight supported on her left leg and the cane, have her move her right leg forward ahead of the cane. If she does this correctly, her heel will be slightly beyond the tip of the cane.

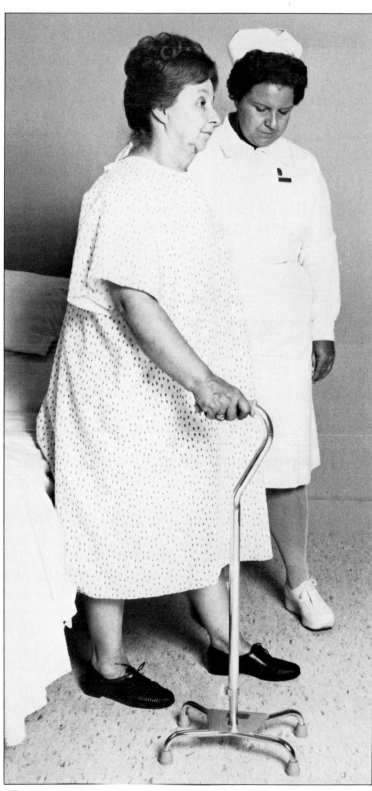

4 Tell Mrs. Samuels to support her weight on her right leg and the cane. Then, have her move her left foot forward, parallel with the cane, as shown in this photo.

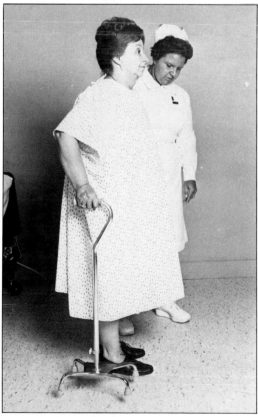

6 Tell Mrs. Samuels to move her left foot forward so it's even with her right foot, as shown. Then, instruct her to move her cane forward as instructed in step 3. Guide her through the above procedure several times until you both feel she's ready to try it alone.

When Mrs. Samuels' family comes to visit, acquaint them with the proper procedure for cane-walking.

Document all patient teaching, along with your patient's progress, in your nurses' notes.

Crutches, canes, and walkers

How to walk with two canes

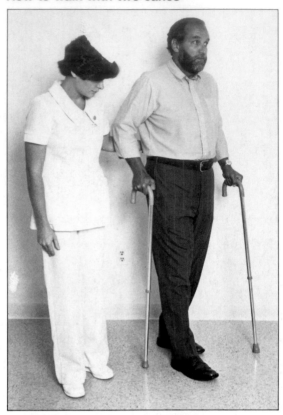

Consider this situation: The physical therapist has started teaching your patient to walk with two canes. You're asked to help your patient practice. Do you know what to do?

First, make sure both canes are the proper size for your patient. Then, review what the physical therapist has taught him. Stand behind your patient and slightly to his side. If necessary, use a transfer belt to steady him, or use his trousers belt.

As you know, your patient will be using either a two-point or a four-point gait. Follow the same procedure you taught for crutch-walking (see pages 105 to 107). Guide your patient until you're both certain he's ready to try it alone.

Getting in and out of a chair with a cane

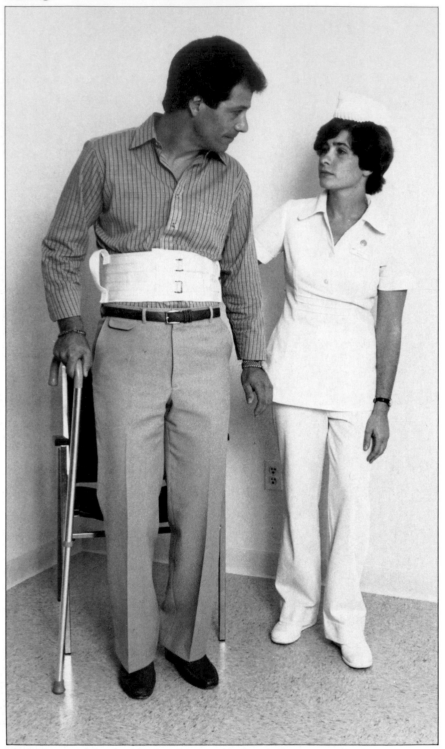

1 *After showing your patient how to walk with a cane, teach him how to get in and out of a chair with it. Follow these guidelines if you're using a chair with armrests:*

First, explain the procedure to your patient. Place a transfer belt around his waist. Instruct him to steady himself with his cane as he stands with the backs of his legs against the chair's seat.

2 You'll stand by his weak side. Then, tell him to move his cane out from his side and reach back with both hands to grasp the chair's armrests.

Have your patient support his weight on the armrests and lower himself onto the seat. Then, instruct him to hook the cane on the armrest or chair back.

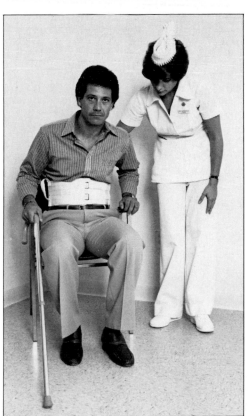

4 Next, have him place his strong foot slightly forward.

Instruct him to lean slightly forward and push against the armrests to raise himself upright.

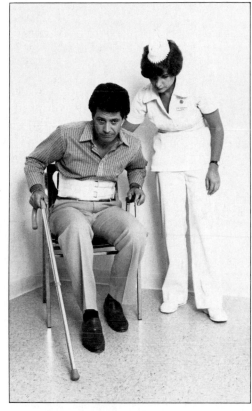

3 Now, teach your patient how to get out of the chair. To do this, stand by his weak side. Instruct him to unhook the cane from the armrest or chair back and hold it in his strong hand, as he grasps the armrests.

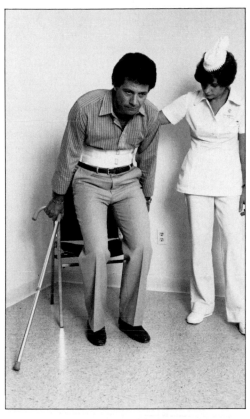

5 Remind him to steady himself by placing the cane's tip about 4" (10 cm) to the side of his strong foot.

Guide your patient as he gets in and out of the chair until you're both certain he's ready to try it alone.

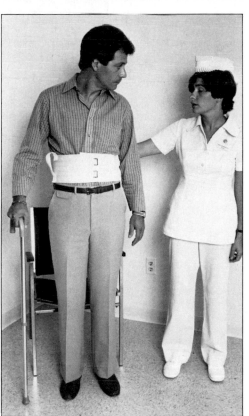

Crutches, canes, and walkers

How to go up and down stairs with a cane

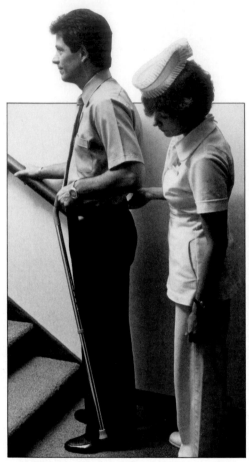

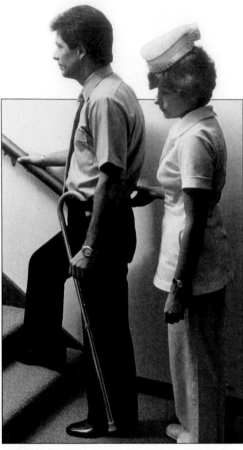

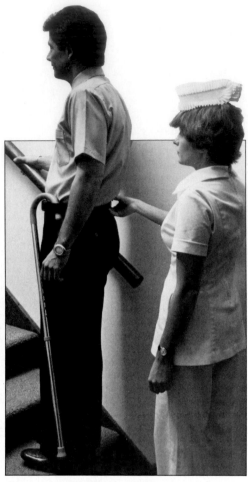

1 *After Mr. Gavin learns how to walk on a flat surface with a cane, show him how to go up and down stairs. As you know, Mr. Gavin has left-sided hemiparesis. With a sturdy banister on both sides of the stairs, here's how to proceed:*

First, explain the procedure to Mr. Gavin and reassure him. Make sure the stairs are safe, clean, dry, and well lighted. Since Mr. Gavin is already wearing a belt, you won't have to place a transfer belt around his waist.

Then, instruct Mr. Gavin to stand at the bottom of the stairs, with his feet about 6″ (15 cm) apart. Make sure his strong side is next to the banister. Have him grasp the banister with his right hand about 4″ (10 cm) from the end. As he does, tell him to transfer his cane to his left hand. Then, instruct him to hook the cane over his arm or belt.

Note: If your patient's using a broad-based cane, tell him to place the cane on the step ahead of him, so his hand's free to grasp the banister.

2 Now, stand behind and slightly to the left of your patient. Grasp his belt to help support him. Do this until you're both certain he can go up and down stairs alone. Remind your patient to look ahead, not at his feet.

Instruct Mr. Gavin to hold onto the banister firmly as he shifts his weight to his left leg. Tell him to pull himself forward with his right hand, using the banister, as he lifts his right foot to the first step.

3 Have him shift his weight to his right leg. Then, instruct him to use the banister to pull himself forward with his right hand as he lifts his left foot to the first step.

Continue guiding your patient through this procedure until he's reached the top of the stairs.

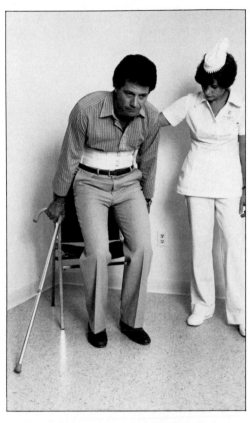

2 You'll stand by his weak side. Then, tell him to move his cane out from his side and reach back with both hands to grasp the chair's armrests.

Have your patient support his weight on the armrests and lower himself onto the seat. Then, instruct him to hook the cane on the armrest or chair back.

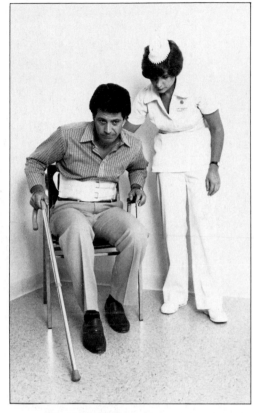

4 Next, have him place his strong foot slightly forward.

Instruct him to lean slightly forward and push against the armrests to raise himself upright.

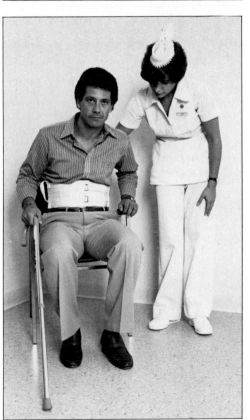

3 Now, teach your patient how to get out of the chair. To do this, stand by his weak side. Instruct him to unhook the cane from the armrest or chair back and hold it in his strong hand, as he grasps the armrests.

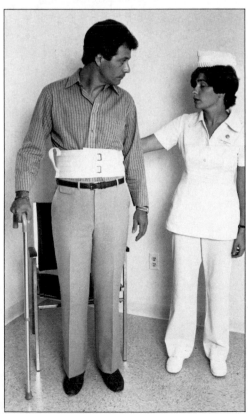

5 Remind him to steady himself by placing the cane's tip about 4" (10 cm) to the side of his strong foot.

Guide your patient as he gets in and out of the chair until you're both certain he's ready to try it alone.

Crutches, canes, and walkers

How to go up and down stairs with a cane

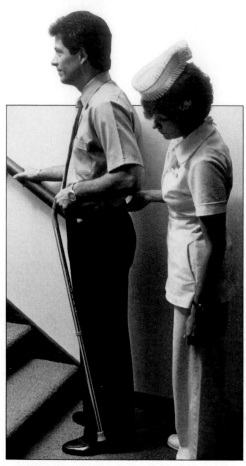

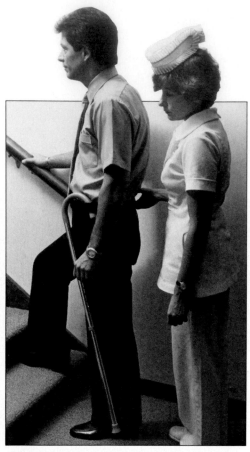

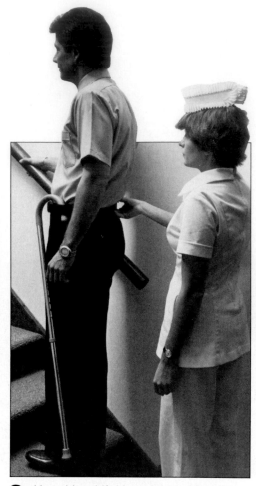

1 *After Mr. Gavin learns how to walk on a flat surface with a cane, show him how to go up and down stairs. As you know, Mr. Gavin has left-sided hemiparesis. With a sturdy banister on both sides of the stairs, here's how to proceed:*

First, explain the procedure to Mr. Gavin and reassure him. Make sure the stairs are safe, clean, dry, and well lighted. Since Mr. Gavin is already wearing a belt, you won't have to place a transfer belt around his waist.

Then, instruct Mr. Gavin to stand at the bottom of the stairs, with his feet about 6″ (15 cm) apart. Make sure his strong side is next to the banister. Have him grasp the banister with his right hand about 4″ (10 cm) from the end. As he does, tell him to transfer his cane to his left hand. Then, instruct him to hook the cane over his arm or belt.

Note: If your patient's using a broad-based cane, tell him to place the cane on the step ahead of him, so his hand's free to grasp the banister.

2 Now, stand behind and slightly to the left of your patient. Grasp his belt to help support him. Do this until you're both certain he can go up and down stairs alone. Remind your patient to look ahead, not at his feet.

Instruct Mr. Gavin to hold onto the banister firmly as he shifts his weight to his left leg. Tell him to pull himself forward with his right hand, using the banister, as he lifts his right foot to the first step.

3 Have him shift his weight to his right leg. Then, instruct him to use the banister to pull himself forward with his right hand as he lifts his left foot to the first step.

Continue guiding your patient through this procedure until he's reached the top of the stairs.

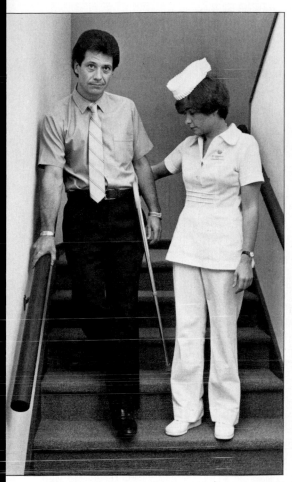

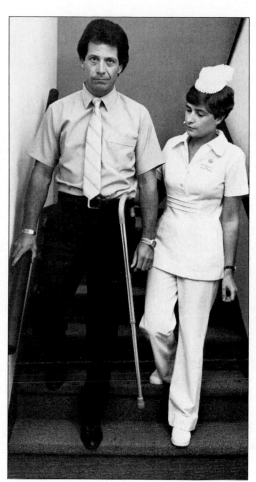

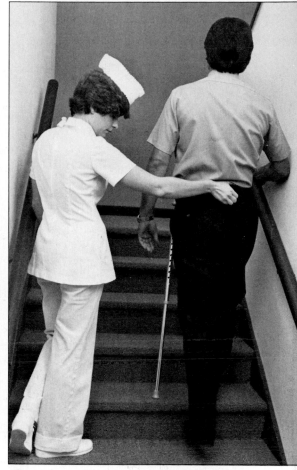

4 Now, help Mr. Gavin turn around and go down the stairs, following the same procedure as above. But, this time, you'll guide him by standing *in front of him,* slightly to his left.

Have your patient lower his *left* foot, then his right foot, to each step. Instruct him to grasp the banister with his right hand to balance himself. Continue to support and encourage him.

5 If Mr. Gavin's going *up* stairs with only one banister on his *left* side, he'll have to go up the stairs backwards. Instruct him to stand with his back to the stairs and his right side next to the banister. Again, stand *in front of him,* slightly to his left. Instruct him to lift his *right* foot, then his left, to each step, following the procedure previously described.

6 Suppose Mr. Gavin's going *downstairs* with only one banister on his *left* side. Teach him to go down the stairs backwards. He'll stand with his back to the stairs and his right side next to the banister. Stand behind your patient, slightly to his left. Have him lower his *left* foot, then his right, to each step, following the same procedure.

Crutches, canes, and walkers

Selecting the best walker for your patient

Whether you work in a hospital or a nursing home, sooner or later you'll have to go to central supply to get a walker for your patient. If you don't have a physical therapist to help you, will you know which type of walker to select? If you're unsure, consider the following:

• Will my patient's diagnosis and prognosis require a special type of walker? A patient with overall muscular weakness, for example, may need a reciprocal walker. If your patient travels extensively, he'll require a collapsible walker.

• How do I know if the walker is the proper height? To determine this, ask your patient to stand between the walker's rear legs, holding the hand grips. The walker should extend from the floor to his hip joint. His elbows should flex about 30°.

• Does the walker you're considering have rubber tips on its legs to prevent slipping? Examine the tips carefully to make sure they're intact. Replace them, if needed.

Note: If your patient has a special problem, you may want to contact a walker manufacturer about special walker features.

Now, carefully study the accompanying chart to familiarize yourself with some of the most common types of walkers. We've also included some helpful hints on proper use.

Stationary

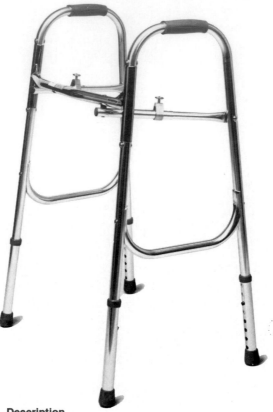

Description

• A metal frame with hand grips, four legs, and no movable parts; usually lightweight and inexpensive
• Some models fold up for travel and easy storage.
• Some models have small front wheels.
• Height is usually adjustable, from 27″ to 37″ (68.5 to 94 cm).

Nursing considerations

• Recommend this type for a patient with good arm strength and balance.
• Teach the patient a three-point or a three-point-and-one gait, as ordered by the doctor or physical therapist.
• If your patient can't lift this walker, recommend one with small front wheels.
  Note: Remind a patient using this walker to advance the front wheels slowly. This will help prevent him from losing his balance.

Rolling

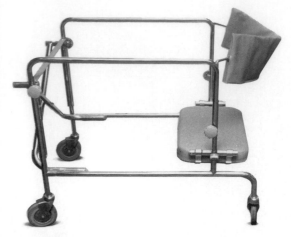

Description

• A metal frame with four legs on wheels; usually expensive
• Available with attached seat
• Available in adjustable heights

Nursing considerations

• Check with a doctor or physical therapist before recommending a rolling walker. These walkers are hazardous for patients lacking balance and coordination.
• If the doctor or physical therapist recommends a rolling walker with a seat for your patient, make sure the seat's the proper height.
• When seated, your patient's hips and knees should flex about 90°.
• Instruct your patient to propel this walker with his legs.

Reciprocal

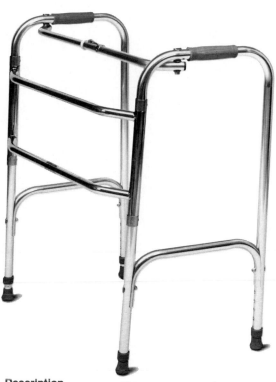

Description

• A metal frame with hand grips, four legs, and a hinge mechanism, allowing one side to be advanced ahead of the other
• Some models fold up for travel and storage.
• Height is usually adjustable from 27" to 37" (68.5 to 94 cm).
• More stable than stationary walker

Nursing considerations

• Recommend this type for a patient with decreased arm strength and balance.
• Teach the patient a two-point or four-point gait, as ordered by the doctor or physical therapist.

Reciprocal walkers: How to teach your patient the two-point gait

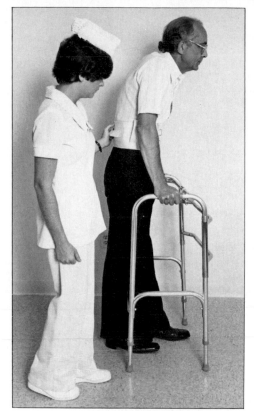

1 *Preparing to teach your patient how to use the two-point gait with a reciprocal walker? Begin by explaining the procedure to him and placing a transfer belt around his waist.*

Then, instruct your patient to stand with his weight evenly distributed between his legs and the walker. Stand behind him, slightly to one side.

Tell him to simultaneously advance the walker's right side and his left foot.

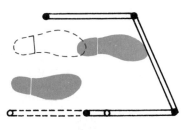

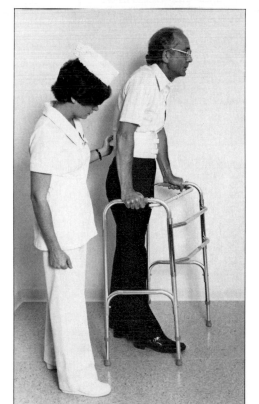

2 Next, have your patient advance the walker's left side and his right foot. Tell him to continue in this manner. Stay with him until you're both confident he can do it alone.

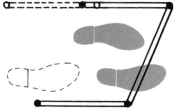

Crutches, canes, and walkers

Reciprocal walkers: How to teach your patient the four-point gait

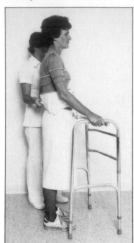

1 *Imagine you want to teach 35-year-old Wilma Vicks how to do the four-point gait with a walker. If you're not sure how to proceed, follow these guidelines carefully:*

First, explain the procedure to Ms. Vicks, and place a transfer belt around her waist. Ask her to evenly distribute her weight between her legs and the walker. In this photostory, the patient's using a Lumex Walk-a-matic reciprocal walker. Stand behind her and slightly to one side.

Then ask your patient to move the right side of the walker forward.

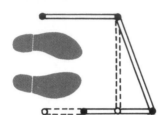

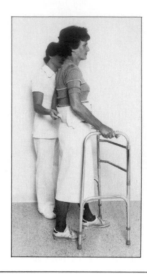

2 Now, tell Ms. Vicks to move her left foot forward.

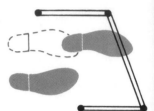

Stationary walker: How to teach your patient the three-point gait (non-weight–bearing)

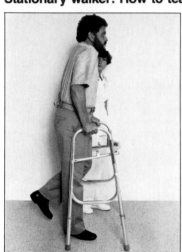

1 *Let's assume you're caring for 42-year-old George James, who's recovering from surgery on his left hip. The doctor has asked you to teach Mr. James the three-point gait with a walker. Do you know how? Study these steps carefully:*

First, explain the procedure to Mr. James, and place a transfer belt around his waist, or use his trousers belt, if he's wearing one. Then, ask him to stand with the walker in front of him. Have him distribute his weight evenly between the walker and his right leg.

Stand behind your patient, slightly to his left side.

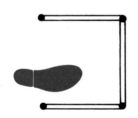

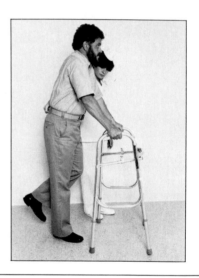

Stationary walker: How to teach your patient the three-point-and-one gait (partial-weight–bearing)

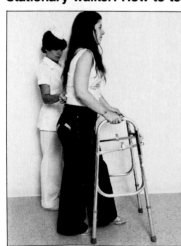

1 *Marion Thisey, a 24-year-old fabric designer, is recovering from surgery on her left leg. The doctor asks you to teach Ms. Thisey the three-point-and-one gait with a walker. Do you know how? Proceed as follows to help a patient with a weak left leg.*

First, explain the procedure to Ms. Thisey, and place a transfer belt around her waist. Then, ask her to stand with the walker positioned slightly in front of her. She'll need to distribute most of her weight between her right leg and the walker, although she should try to support some weight on her left leg.

Stand behind Ms. Thisey and slightly to her side. Then, instruct her to shift all her weight to her right leg as she lifts and advances the walker and her left leg as far as 8″ (20 cm).

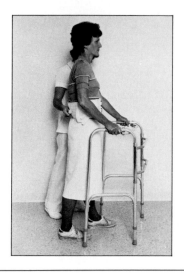

3 Instruct your patient to move the left side of the walker forward.

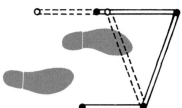

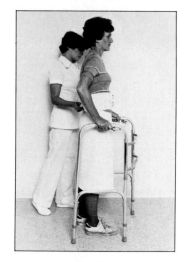

4 Have her move her right foot forward.
Encourage her to repeat the procedure. Stay with her until you're both certain she can use the walker correctly without assistance.

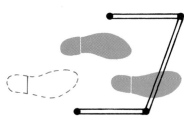

2 Now, instruct Mr. James to shift his weight to his right leg, as he lifts and advances the walker approximately 8″ (20 cm).

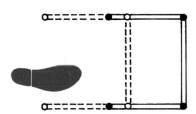

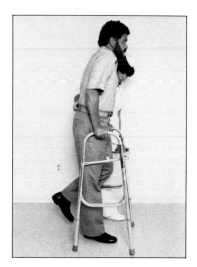

3 Then, have him swing his right leg about 8″ (20 cm) forward, as he supports his weight on the walker. Remind him not to put any weight on his left leg.
Tell him to repeat these steps—moving first the walker, then his right leg. Stay with him until you're both confident he can do it alone.

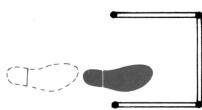

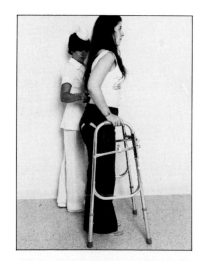

2 Next, tell your patient to shift her weight to her left leg and the walker. As she does, instruct her to move her right leg as far as 8″ (20 cm) forward.
Encourage Ms. Thisey to repeat this procedure—moving first her left leg (and the walker), then the other. Continue to guide her through these steps until you're both certain she can do it alone.
To show your patient how to get in and out of a chair using a walker, see page 128.

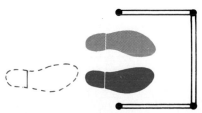

Crutches, canes, and walkers

Getting in and out of a chair with a walker

1 *Now you want to show George James how to get in and out of a chair with a walker. Using a chair with armrests, here's the procedure to follow:*

First, explain the procedure to your patient. Place a transfer belt around his waist, or grasp his trousers belt, as the nurse is doing here. Then, instruct Mr. James to stand so his right leg is against the front of the chair seat. His left leg should be slightly off the floor. Ask your patient to position the walker in front of him.

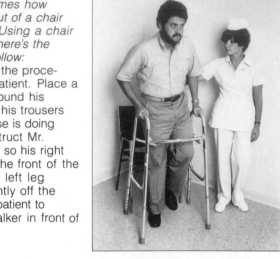

2 Ask Mr. James to grasp the left armrest of the chair with his left hand. Have him shift his weight to his left hand and right leg, then grasp the other armrest with his right hand.

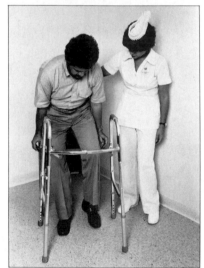

3 Now, instruct your patient to lower himself onto the chair seat and slide back. Have him place the walker beside the chair.

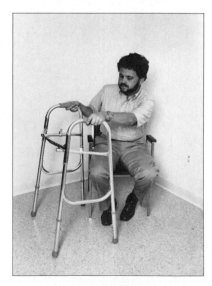

4 Now, teach Mr. James to get out of the chair. First, instruct him to position the walker in front of him and slide forward in the chair. Have him position his right leg against the seat and his left leg forward, as shown here.

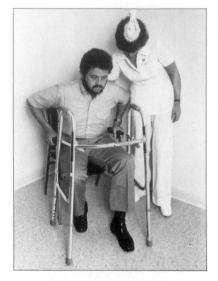

5 Next, tell him to push his hands against the armrests and raise himself out of the seat. Supporting his weight with his left hand and right leg, instruct him to grasp the walker's right hand grip with his right hand.

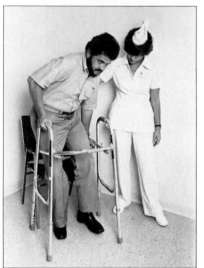

6 Tell Mr. James to raise himself to a standing position. As he does, he'll use his left hand to grasp the left hand grip.

Finally, have him distribute his weight between his hands and right foot. He can now start to use the walker.

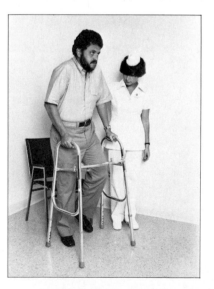

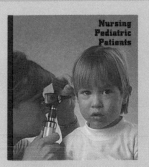
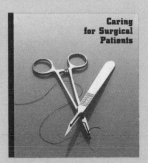
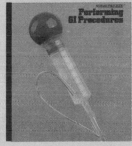
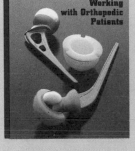
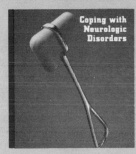
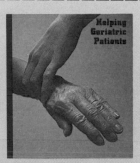
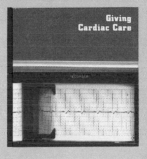
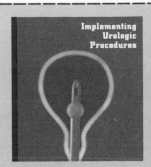
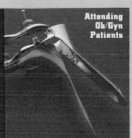
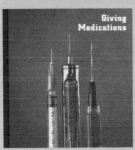

© 1983 Intermed Communications, Inc.

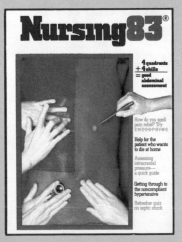

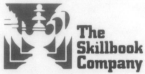
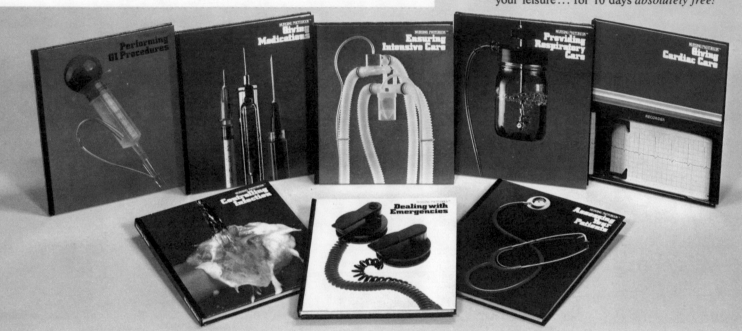

Wheelchairs

What's the proper wheelchair for your patient?

Sure, you probably know a lot about wheelchairs. But do you know how to select or recommend the proper wheelchair for your patient? For example, do you know which wheelchair features to select for a patient with a leg amputation, hemiplegia, or cerebral palsy?

Or, do you know:
• how to operate a power-driven wheelchair?
• how to lock a lever brake?
• how to remove an armrest?

In this section we'll answer these questions. We'll also include some special guidelines and considerations. Read the material thoroughly.

If you're recommending or selecting a wheelchair for your patient, familiarize yourself with various wheelchair sizes and styles. Learn which one is right for your patient. To do this, first compare your patient's measurements with the wheelchair's dimensions to determine the size wheelchair he'll need. As you know, wheelchairs come in three sizes: *standard adult, intermediate or junior* (for small adults and older children), and *child* (for children up to age 6).

However, to ensure your patient's safety and comfort, you'll also want to consider the width of the seat and the height from the floor, the height of the back and armrests, the length of the legrests, and whether the legrests and armrests are removable.

Determine how your patient's condition will affect the wheelchair he needs and how he'll propel it.
• Consider his diagnosis and prognosis—whether his condition might deteriorate or improve. For example, if he has progressive muscular dystrophy, he may eventually have upper body weakness—he'll need a wheelchair with a semireclining back or a higher backrest.
• If your patient has bilateral leg amputations, recommend a chair with wheels set back a few inches. Because your patient's center of gravity will be near his chest, instead of his pelvis, he'll need this type wheelchair to prevent the chair from tipping.
• If your patient has a below-the-knee amputation, edema, or a newly applied cast, suggest a wheelchair with legrests that can be elevated.
• If your patient has use of both arms, recommend a two-arm drive wheelchair.
• If he has use of just one arm, advise your patient to get a one-arm drive wheelchair.
• For a patient with poor sitting balance, recommend a chair with a solid seat rather than a collapsible one.

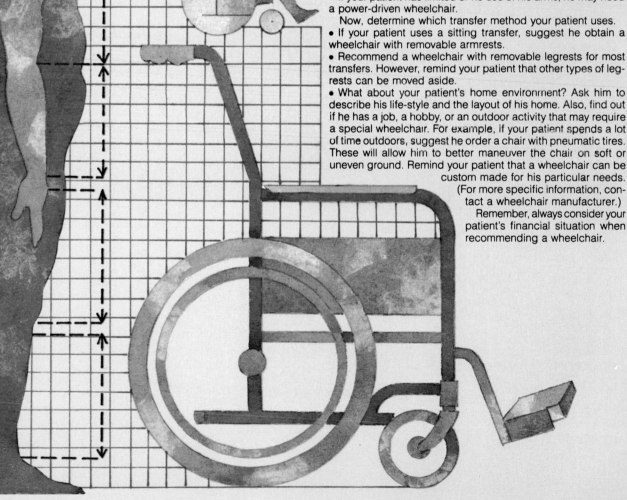

• If your patient has arm or hand weakness, suggest he use a wheelchair with one of several types of hand projections on the handrims. Hand projections will allow your patient to grasp the handrims more firmly.
• If your patient has limited or no use of his arms, he may need a power-driven wheelchair.

Now, determine which transfer method your patient uses.
• If your patient uses a sitting transfer, suggest he obtain a wheelchair with removable armrests.
• Recommend a wheelchair with removable legrests for most transfers. However, remind your patient that other types of legrests can be moved aside.
• What about your patient's home environment? Ask him to describe his life-style and the layout of his home. Also, find out if he has a job, a hobby, or an outdoor activity that may require a special wheelchair. For example, if your patient spends a lot of time outdoors, suggest he order a chair with pneumatic tires. These will allow him to better maneuver the chair on soft or uneven ground. Remind your patient that a wheelchair can be custom made for his particular needs. (For more specific information, contact a wheelchair manufacturer.)

Remember, always consider your patient's financial situation when recommending a wheelchair.

Wheelchairs

Understanding wheelchair basics

Before teaching your patient how to use his wheelchair, you'll want to familiarize yourself with wheelchair basics. To learn how each part works and how to use the special features properly, study this chart carefully.

Handrims

Nursing considerations
• Hand projections are recommended for patients with decreased hand and arm strength.
• To propel a wheelchair with hand projections forward, have your patient grasp the projections and push them away from him. To move the chair backward, tell your patient to grasp the projections and pull them toward him.
• Be sure to consider how far hand projections protrude when measuring a wheelchair for use in a patient's home. Make sure they'll fit through doorways and hallways.

Wheelchair feature
Two-arm drive

Description
A handrim lies near each wheel. The right handrim moves the right wheel; the left handrim moves the left wheel. May have hand projections.

How to use
To propel a wheelchair with two-arm drive forward or backward, move both handrims simultaneously. To turn to the left, move the right handrim only. To turn to the right, move the left handrim only.

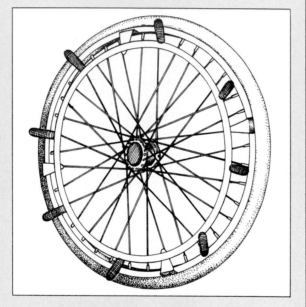

Wheelchair feature
One-arm drive

Description
Two handrims, one smaller than the other, lie near one wheel. The outer, smaller rim moves the opposite wheel. The inner, larger rim moves the closest wheel. May have hand projections.

How to use
To propel a wheelchair with one-arm drive, move both handrims with one hand. To turn left or right, move the appropriate handrim.

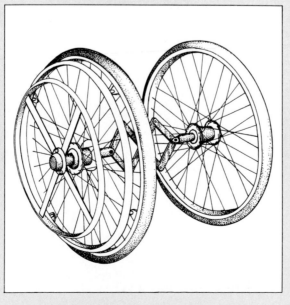

Brake

Nursing considerations
• Remember to lock wheels before beginning transfer.

Wheelchair feature
Toggle

Description
Toggle lever locks projection against the wheel to keep it from moving.

How to use
Push toggle lever forward to lock the projection against the wheel. Pull the lever back to release the brake.

Wheelchair feature
Lever

Description
Lever fits into a series of notches, regulating the amount of pressure put against the wheel by the projection.

How to use
Slide brake lever into the notch farthest from the wheel for maximum pressure. To release the brake, slide the lever into the notch closest to the wheel.
• Remind your patient to use the intermediate notches on the lever brake to regulate his wheelchair speed when he's going down an incline.

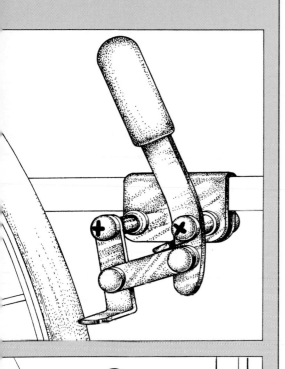

Armrests

Nursing considerations

If your patient's being moved using a transfer board, make sure his wheelchair has removable armrests.

• Advise patient to hang detached armrest on wheelchair during transfer.

• Make sure armrests are 1″ (2.5 cm) higher than the distance from the wheelchair's seat to the patient's elbow.

• Special armrests can be ordered to fit specific patient needs; for example, armrests with a lowered front portion to allow a wheelchair to slide close to a table or desk.

Wheelchair feature
Removable

Description
Armrests detach from the chair when the lock's released.

How to use
Simultaneously, release the lock and lift armrest.

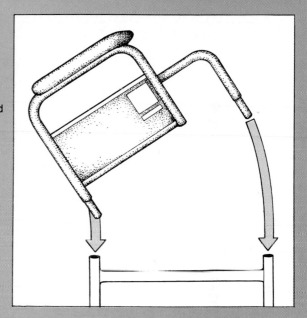

Wheelchair feature
Stationary

Description
Armrests stay in place and may be padded for comfort.

How to use
Adjust height for patient comfort.

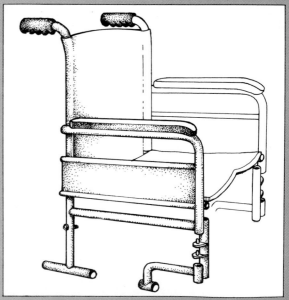

Wheelchairs

Understanding wheelchair basics continued

Legrests

Nursing considerations
• Removable or swing-away legrests are preferred for all transfers.
• If your patient's transferring to a wheelchair with stationary legrests, instruct him to flip up the foot pedals and position the chair as close to the bed as possible.
• Make sure leg pads lie directly behind your patient's calves.
• Adjust legrest length so the back of the patient's knee is approximately 1" (2.5 cm) above the seat. This prevents pressure on the popliteal area.
• To prevent tipping, caution a patient using a chair with elevated legrests not to lean forward. Instruct him to carry any parcels on the back of the wheelchair and to lean to the side of the wheelchair when he's picking something up from the floor.
• If your patient has bilateral leg amputations, make sure the wheelchair's footrests are weighted.
• If your patient has a below-the-knee amputation, instruct him to prevent flexion contractures of the knee by securing a padded board (with knee extension) to his wheelchair seat, instead of an elevating legrest.

Wheelchair feature
Swing-away

Description
Legrests swing away from the front of the wheelchair for easy access.

How to use
Release the lock and swing the legrests outward and to the rear.

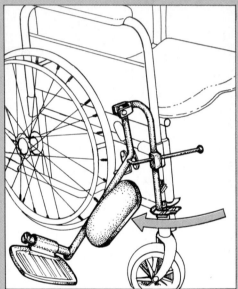
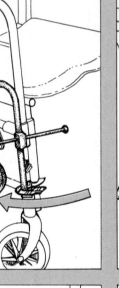

Wheelchair feature
Stationary

Description
Foot pedals and leg pads flip to the side.

How to use
Turn the leg pads to the side and flip up the foot pedals.

Wheelchair feature
Removable

Description
Legrests swing to the side and lift off.

How to use
Release the lock, swing the legrests outward and to the rear. Then, lift them off.

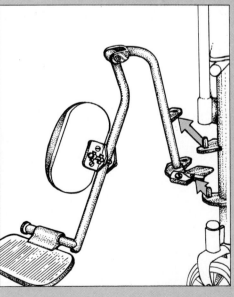

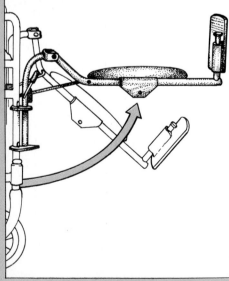

Wheelchair feature
Elevating

Description
Legrests lift up so they're horizontal with the seat.

How to use
Raise legrests to appropriate height and angle. Lock them in place.

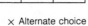

How your patient's condition affects wheelchair selection

As you know, when you select a wheelchair for your patient, you'll have to consider his size and transfer method. But you'll also want to consider his condition and mobility potential. This chart shows some of the wheelchair features available and how you can combine them to meet your patient's needs.

		Hemiplegia	Paraplegia	Quadriplegia	Cerebral palsy	Arthritis	Bilateral amputation
TYPE	**Standard**	⊗	⊗	⊗	⊗	⊗	
	Motorized			×			
	Special	×				×	⊗
HANDRIMS	**Standard**	⊗	⊗	⊗	⊗	⊗	⊗
	One-arm drive	×		×			
	Pegs or knobs			×	×	×	
BRAKES	**Toggle**	×	×	⊗	⊗	⊗	×
	Lever	×	⊗		×		⊗
	Brake extension	⊗		×		×	
	Special	×		×			
BACK	**Fixed**	⊗	⊗		⊗	⊗	⊗
	Reclining			⊗	×	×	
	Head extension	×	×	⊗	×	×	×
ARMRESTS	**Fixed**	⊗			⊗	⊗	⊗
	Removable		⊗	⊗	×	×	
FOOT- AND LEGRESTS	**Swing-detachable**	⊗	⊗	⊗	⊗	⊗	⊗
	Elevating legrest	×	×	×	×	×	×
	Heel loops	⊗	⊗	⊗	⊗	⊗	⊗
	Toe loops		×	×	×	×	

⊗ Preferred   × Alternate choice

The hows and whys of power-driven wheelchairs

How much do you know about power-driven wheelchairs? If you're like many nurses, you'll probably answer, "Very little."

Although a power-driven wheelchair may be used by any patient using a wheelchair, it is essential for ambulation if your patient has severe arm and hand weakness.

Most power-driven wheelchairs are battery-powered. The battery pack's located at the back of the chair, near the floor. The battery pack must be recharged every night to ensure adequate power for the next day's use.

Power-driven wheelchairs operate in various ways: for example, by a toggle switch, a mouthpiece, or a chin control.

• A wheelchair with a toggle switch is hand-controlled—the patient pushes the switch in the direction he wants to move.

• A wheelchair with a mouthpiece control may be used by a patient with minimal hand strength, such as a quadriplegic. The mouthpiece control attaches to a tube connected to the motor.

The patient directs the wheelchair by blowing into the mouthpiece. (For example, two short puffs may initiate a left turn.)

• A wheelchair with a chin control may also be used by a patient with minimal hand strength. The chin lever attaches to an arm connected to the battery cable. The patient uses his chin to push the lever in the direction he wants to move.

Remember: An operating mechanism and many other special features can be custom designed to meet your patient's needs. Contact a wheelchair manufacturer for more information.

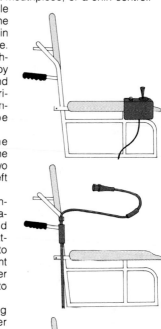

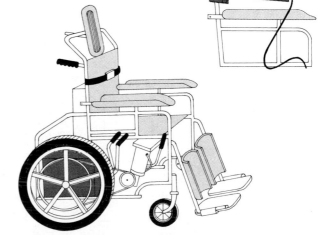

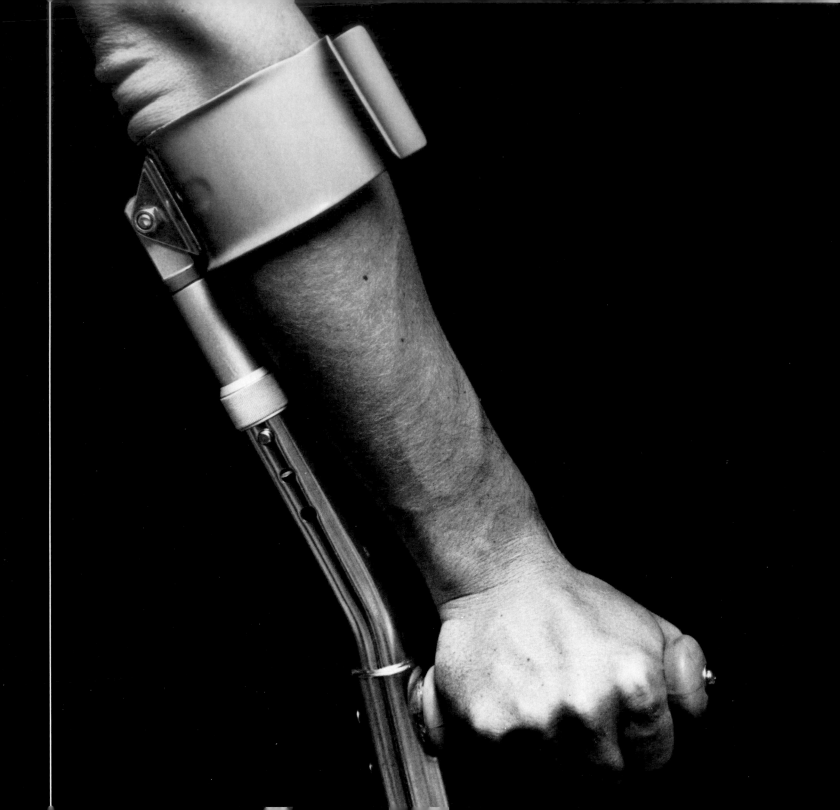

Dealing with Special Situations

Environmental considerations

Environmental considerations

Let's assume your patient's ready to be discharged from the hospital. Do you know how to properly prepare him for any special situations he may encounter? For example, do you know how to teach a patient using crutches, a cane, a walker, or a wheelchair to pick up something from the floor? Or, how to get up from the floor if he falls? Do you know when to recommend a lapboard, adaptive reachers, or a carrying bag?

In this section, we'll answer these questions and give you some addi-tional tips that'll help you improve your patient's emotional outlook. We'll suggest ways you can help your patient adapt to his home after his discharge from the hospital. We'll also give you some fire safety hints you'll want to share with your patient.

For the patient in a wheelchair: Picking up an item from the floor

1 *Let's say you're going to teach your patient how to pick up something from the floor while he's sitting in a wheelchair. Whenever possible, instruct him to do this by leaning to the side of the wheelchair, rather than forward, to avoid falling out. But, make sure your patient has enough arm strength to hold himself in the chair as he grasps the item. Now, follow the guidelines below carefully:*

First, thoroughly explain the procedure to your patient. Place an item, for example, a sweater, on the floor. Have your patient position his wheelchair so his left side's closest to the sweater. Now, instruct him to lock the chair's wheels.

Remember, if your patient has hemiparesis, tell him to always place his strong side closest to the sweater. Then he'll reach with his strong arm.

2 Have your patient grasp the armrest with his right hand as he leans over the side of the wheelchair to pick up the sweater with his left hand, as shown in this photo.

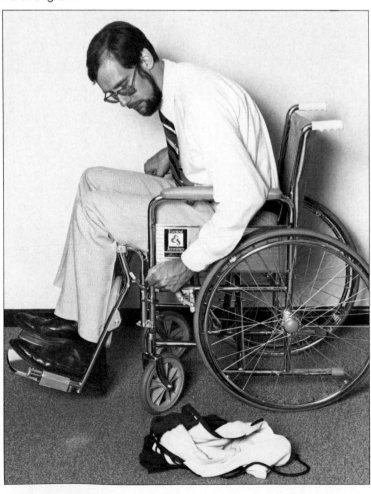

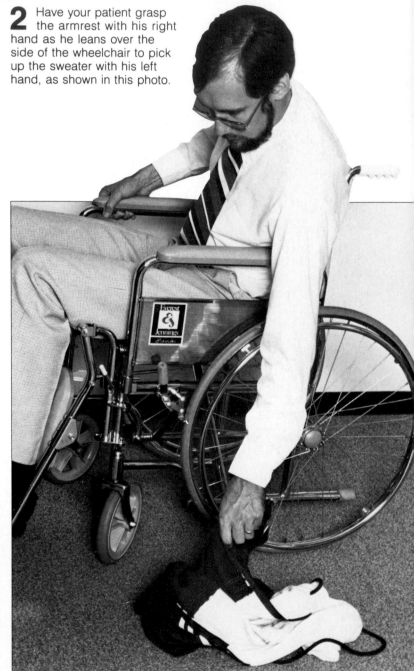

3 If your patient has upper-body weakness or poor balance, and can't hold onto the armrest, recommend he hook his wrist or elbow around the armrest as he leans over the side of the wheelchair to pick up the sweater with his other hand.

Or, suggest he use a reacher.

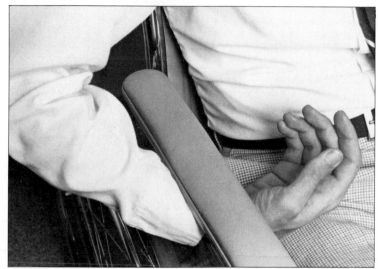

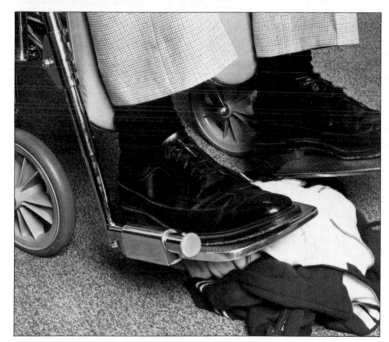

4 Suppose your patient doesn't have a reacher and can't pick up the sweater by leaning over the side of the wheelchair. Show him how to pick it up by leaning forward in the wheelchair.

To do this, instruct your patient to position the wheelchair so the sweater's about midway between the casters.

The wheelchair's casters should face forward, as shown in this photo.

Important: Never recommend this method to a patient with poor arm strength, a displaced center of gravity (such as a patient with a leg cast), or a patient who can't position both feet flat on the floor.

5 Next, tell your patient to lock the chair's wheels and push the foot pedals up. Have him place his feet flat on the floor and grasp the armrest with his right hand. He'll lean forward in the chair and use his left hand to pick up the sweater, as shown here.

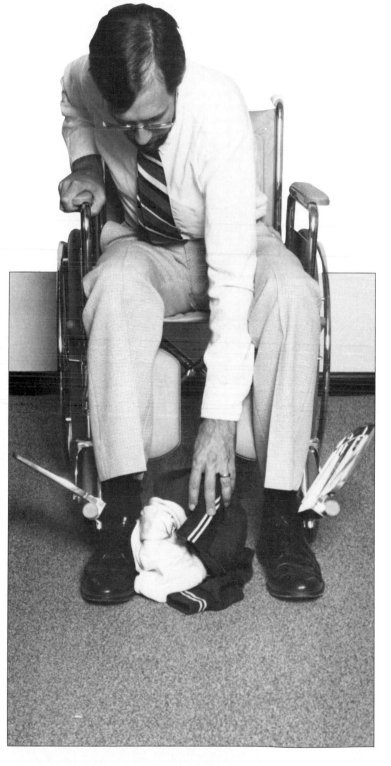

Environmental considerations

Teaching a crutch-walking patient to pick up an item from the floor

1 *Jeff Bardos, a 20-year-old student, has recently had knee surgery and is walking with crutches. But as he walks down the hall you see him drop a magazine. Show him the proper way to pick up the magazine from the floor. Here's how:*

First, carefully explain the procedure to Jeff. Then, instruct him to look around the room for a low piece of furniture, for example, a chair. Now, have him push the magazine over to the chair with his foot or one crutch, as shown here.

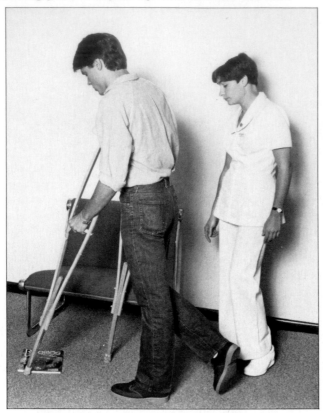

2 Tell Jeff to shift his crutches to one hand and sit down in the chair, following the procedure described on pages 112 to 113.

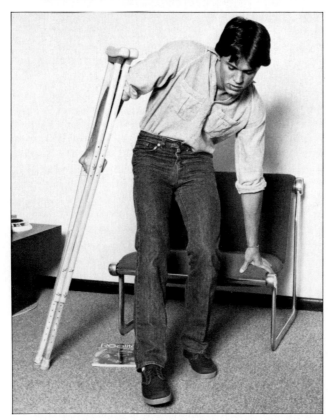

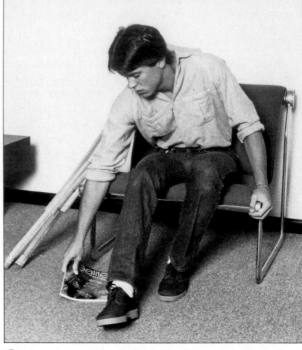

3 Next, have your patient lean his crutches against the chair and steady himself with one hand. Then, tell him to lean forward in the chair, reach down, and pick up the magazine with his other hand.

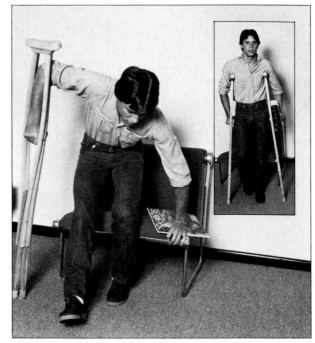

4 Now, as Jeff grasps the crutches with his right hand, instruct him to push himself off the chair with his left hand.

[Inset] Finally, tell him to transfer one crutch to his left hand (which is holding the magazine) as he rises.

Showing a patient with a walker how to pick up something from the floor

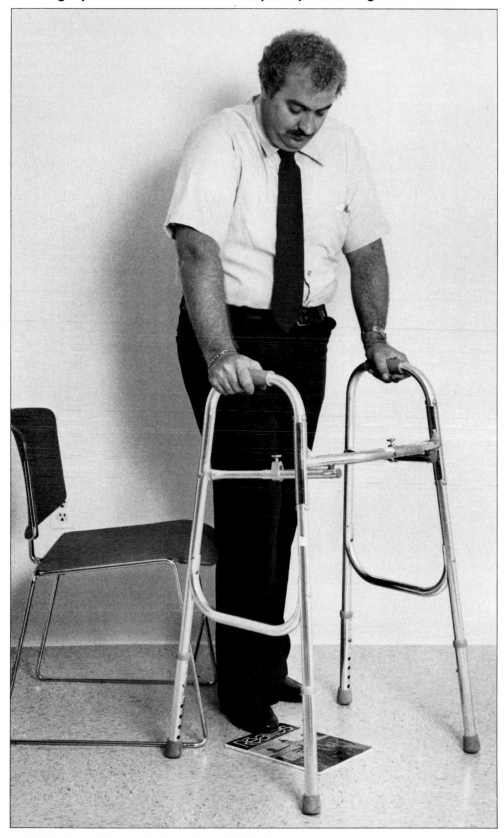

1 *Can you show a patient using a walker how to pick up a magazine from the floor? If you're unsure, follow these guidelines:*

First, explain the procedure to your patient. Then, tell him to look around the room for a low piece of furniture, for example, a chair. Instruct him to use his walker or foot to push the magazine over to the chair, as shown in this photo.

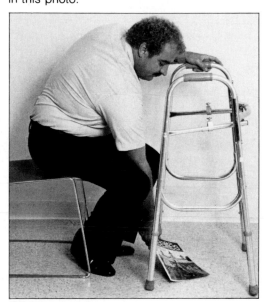

2 Now, ask your patient to sit down in the chair, following the guidelines on page 128. When he's in the chair, instruct him to lean forward and pick up the magazine.

Finally, tell him to support his weight on the walker as he stands up.

Environmental considerations

Coping with falls: The wheelchair patient

1 *If your patient will be using a wheelchair, you'll want to teach him how to deal with some special situations. Begin by showing him how to get back into his wheelchair if he accidentally falls out. To do this, follow these steps:*

First, explain the procedure to your patient. Then, ask a coworker to help you lower your patient to the floor, with his legs extended. When he's on the floor, tell your patient to look around the room for a low, sturdy piece of furniture, for example, a coffee table. He'll need it for support.

Next, instruct your patient to place his hands, palms down, beside his hips. Have him push down with his hands and lift his buttocks off the floor. As he does this, tell him to inch his way toward the wheelchair and grasp the armrest as shown here.

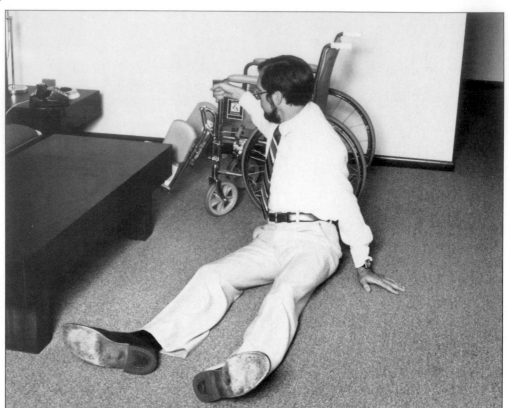

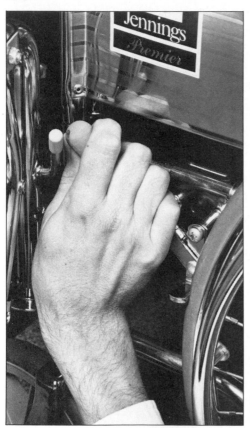

2 Now, he'll unlock the wheelchair's brakes, if necessary. Then, have your patient inch his way over to the table, pushing or pulling the wheelchair with him.

When he reaches the table, instruct your patient to position the wheelchair so the front of the seat is facing the table, as shown in the next photo. Have him lock the wheelchair's brakes and move the legrests out of the way.

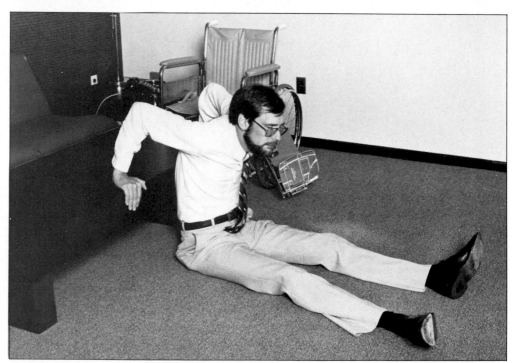

3 Next, tell your patient to position himself with his back toward the table. He must then reach back and place both hands on the table, as shown in this photo. Instruct him to push down and lift his buttocks off the floor onto the table. Then, have him slide back on the table so he's as close as possible to the front of the wheelchair.

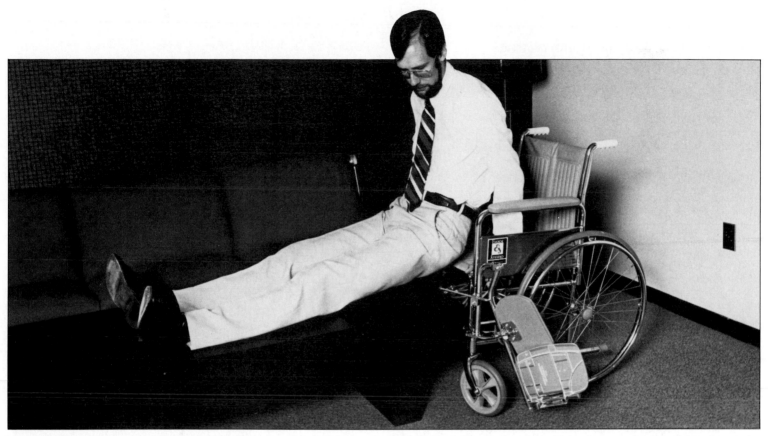

4 Now, ask your patient to reach back and place his hands on the wheelchair's seat. Have him push down with both hands and lift himself onto the chair. Then, he can slide back into the seat and position himself properly.

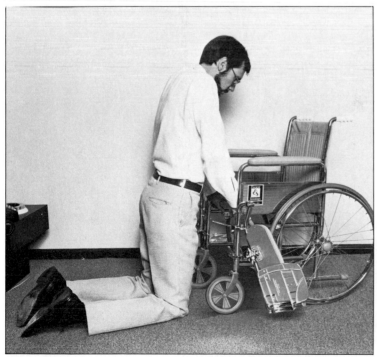

5 Suppose your patient can support his weight on his knees. Tell him to kneel in front of the wheelchair so his chest is toward the seat. Have him place his hands on the seat, as shown here, and push down, lifting himself to seat level.

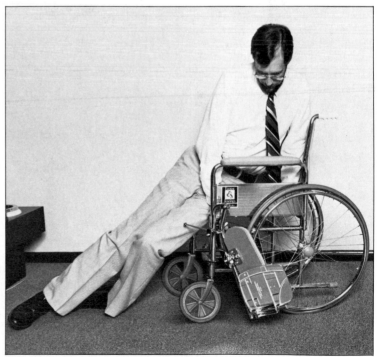

6 Then, tell your patient to support his weight with one hand as he turns his body around and into the seat. When that's accomplished, your patient can slide back in the seat and position himself properly. Document the entire procedure.

Environmental considerations

Coping with falls: The patient with crutches

1 *Now, you'll want to show your patient, Jeff Bardos, how to get up if he falls. To do this, follow these steps:*

First, explain the procedure to your patient. With the help of a coworker, carefully lower him to the floor to simulate a fall. When he's on the floor, have him sit with his legs extended and his hands beside his hips.

Tell Jeff to look around the room for a low, sturdy piece of furniture, for example, a coffee table. Now, instruct your patient to inch backward toward the table by pushing his hands down on the floor and lifting his buttocks up. As he does, he can carry both crutches in one hand.

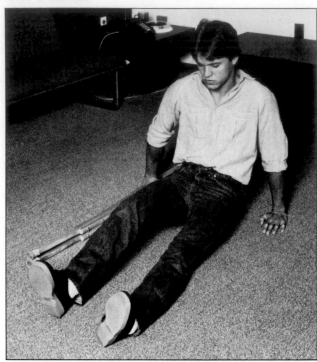

2 When he's next to the table, instruct Jeff to lean his crutches against it. Then, tell him to reach back and place both hands on the table top, as shown here.

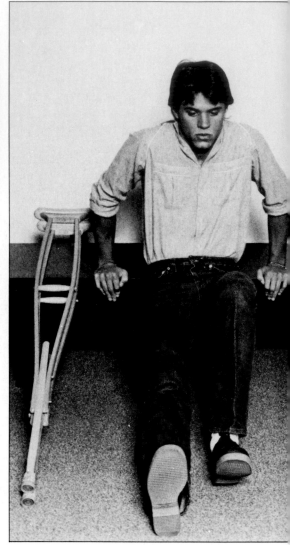

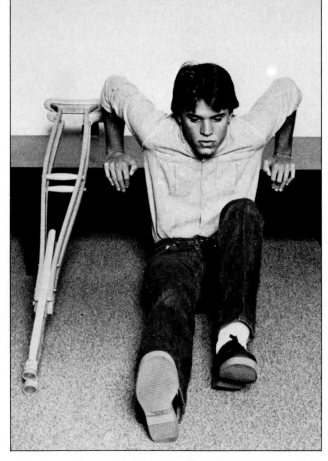

3 Next, ask Jeff to press down on the table top and lift his buttocks onto the table.

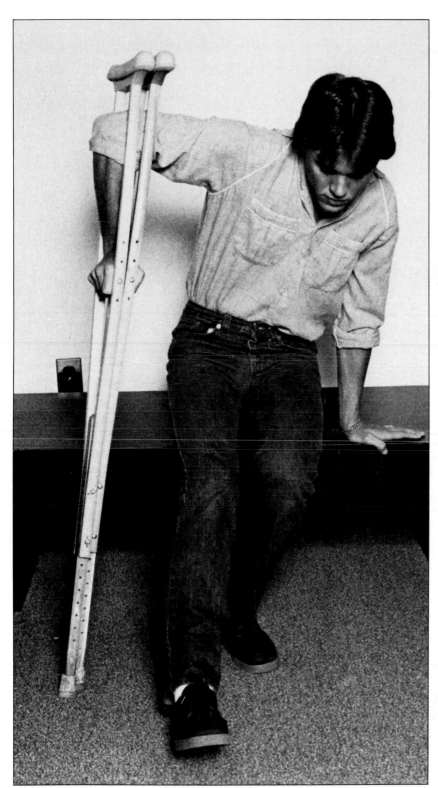

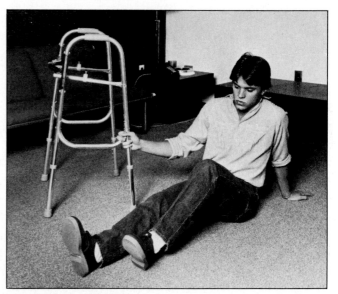

5 But, what if Jeff's using a walker instead of crutches? Show him how to get to his feet, using this method: After explaining the procedure, help lower him to the floor. Then, have him follow the procedure described in step 2 to inch his way to a piece of low, sturdy furniture. He'll pull the walker with one hand.

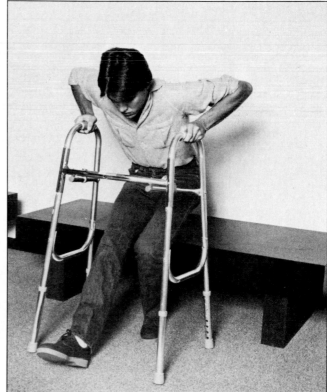

4 Tell him to grasp both crutches in one hand. As he steadies himself with the crutches, have him raise himself to standing position by pushing down with the other hand. After that, he can transfer one of the crutches to his other hand.

6 When your patient gets to the table, instruct him to lift his buttocks onto the table, as described in step 3. Then, he'll position the walker in front of him and raise himself to a standing position.

Environmental considerations

For the wheelchair patient: How to go up and down stairs

1 *Consider this situation: Johanna Corboy, a 38-year-old musician, is paralyzed from the waist down after an automobile accident. The physical therapist has taught Ms. Corboy to use a wheelchair. But, you'll want to show her how to go up and down stairs in a sitting position. Follow this procedure:*

First, thoroughly explain the procedure to Ms. Corboy. Then, instruct her to move her wheelchair over to the stairs and lock the chair's wheels. Tell her to swing the legrests out of the way. Place a footstool in front of the wheelchair so she can rest her legs on it. Have her sit at the edge of the seat, with her hands beside her hips, as shown here.

Remember: If your patient will be using this technique, she'll need someone to carry her wheelchair up or down the stairs for her. Or tell her to keep a second wheelchair upstairs.

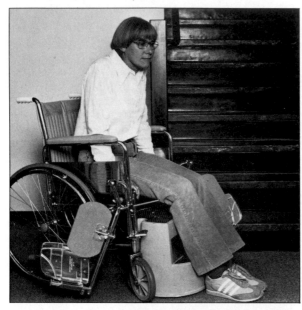

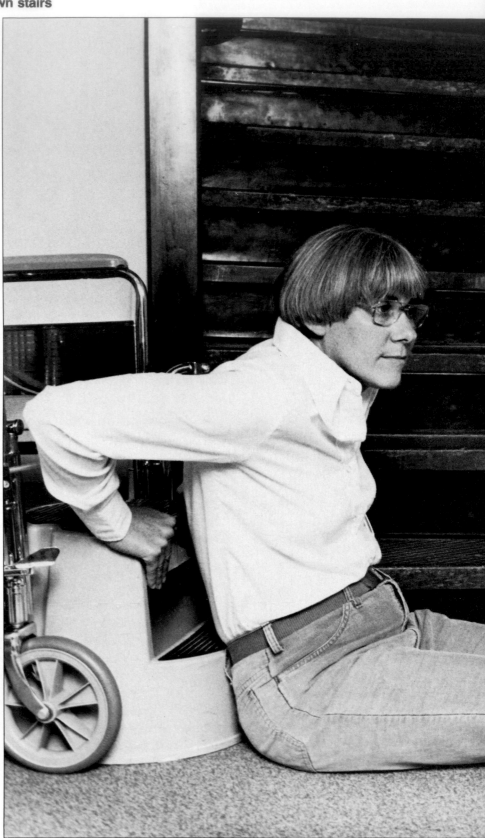

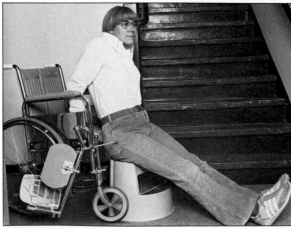

2 Now, tell Ms. Corboy to push her palms against the chair's seat and slowly lower herself to the footstool, as shown here.

3 Then, have her push her hands against the footstool and lower herself to the floor.
Note: If your patient's wheelchair has removable armrests, she can position the chair so the side of the wheelchair is parallel to the stairs. Then, tell her to lift herself directly onto the second or third step.

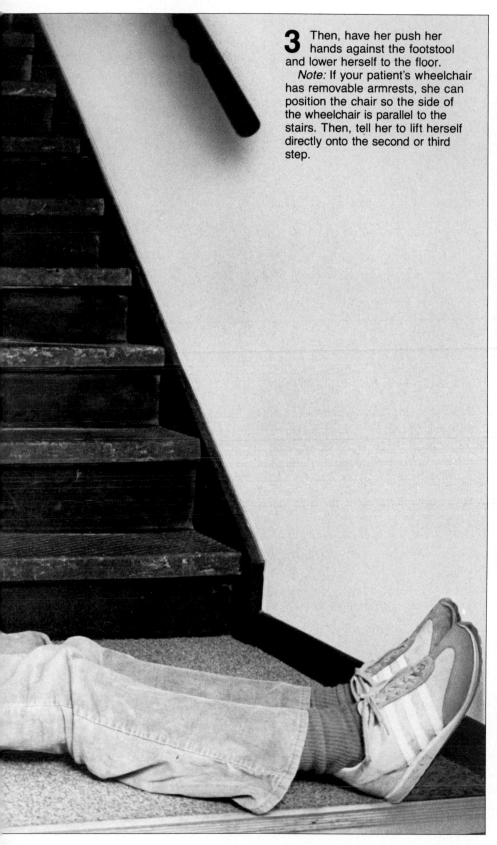

4 Instruct Ms. Corboy to reach back and place her hands on the floor, as shown here. She can then push down and inch herself backward, so her back is toward the stairs.

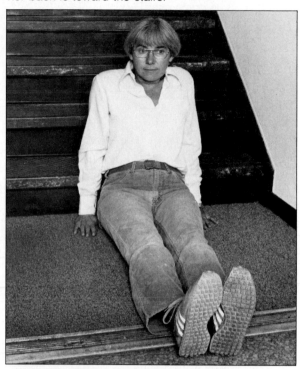

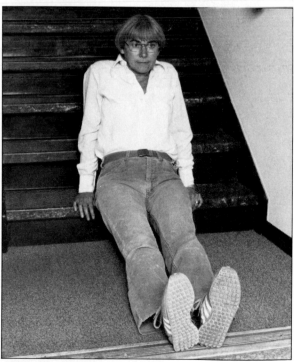

5 Now, tell Ms. Corboy to reach back and place her hands on the first step. Have her push down and lift herself onto the step.

Environmental considerations

For the wheelchair patient: How to go up and down stairs continued

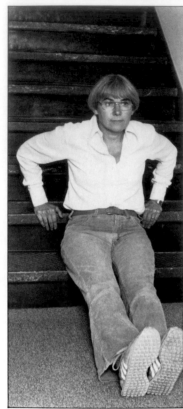

6 Then, instruct your patient to repeat this procedure by pushing down and lifting herself onto the second step. Tell her to continue this procedure until she reaches the top step.

7 After Ms. Corboy takes a short rest, show her how to go down the stairs, facing forward. To do this, have her sit at the edge of the landing, facing forward with her legs extended in front of her. Then, she'll lower her buttocks and her hands, onto each step, as shown here.
☎ *Nursing tip:* To prevent your patient's heels from catching on the steps, have her use her hands to position her legs onto the next lower step, if necessary.

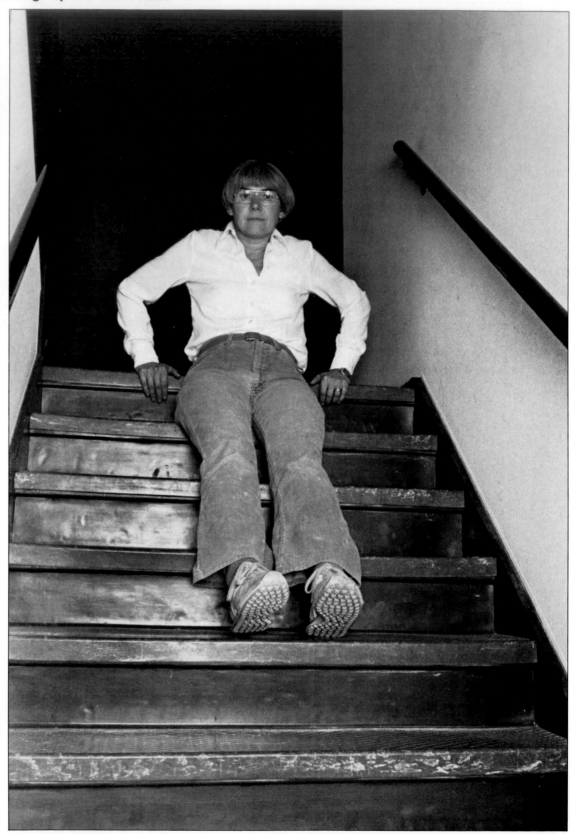

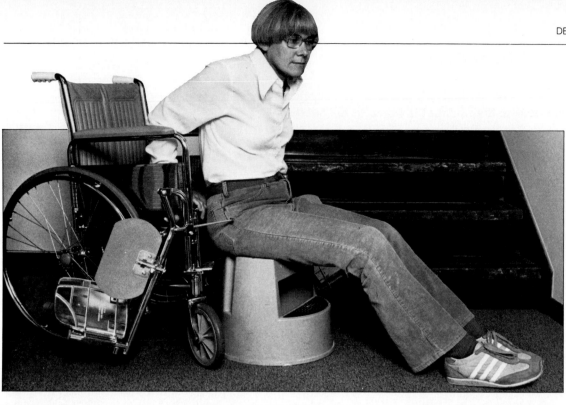

8 When your patient reaches the bottom of the stairs, she'll get back into her wheelchair by lifting herself on the footstool, then to the chair's seat, as described in step 2.

Remind your patient to check the backs of her heels for skin irritation, which may be caused by dragging her heels up the stairs. If skin irritation's present, tell your patient to stop using this stair-climbing method.

Carrying devices

Sooner or later a patient using a wheelchair, crutches, or a walker will have to carry something from one place to another. Depending on the object's size, and your patient's condition and strength, he may want to use a lapboard, basket, knapsack, carrying pouch, or cart with wheels. Before your patient leaves the hospital, you'll want to familiarize him with each of these carrying aids. Also, suggest he buy or rent one of these aids for home use.

Here are some suggestions to keep in mind when recommending any of these aids:
• Is your patient using a wheelchair? If so, a *lapboard* will probably be the most useful carrying aid. When secured to the chair's armrests, the lapboard keeps the object within your patient's reach. It also keeps the object off his lap, which is advantageous if the object's sharp, hot, or heavy.

📨 *Nursing tip:* In some cases, a transfer board can double as a lapboard. If your patient uses a transfer board, have him place the board across the chair's armrests and hold it in place. But, remind your patient that a transfer board won't be as steady as a lapboard, and shouldn't be used to carry hot or awkward items.
• A patient using a wheelchair may want to push a *cart* to transport more than one thing at a time. But, remember, your patient must have good arm strength and balance to push any type of cart.
• A patient using a wheelchair can also carry items in a *canvas, vinyl, or nylon bag* attached to the chair's back with snaps or Velcro straps. (This type of bag can also be attached to a walker.) Also available for walkers and for wheelchairs are various plastic, metal, or wicker *baskets,* which can be hooked or snapped over a walker's metal frame or to a wheelchair's arm.
• If your patient uses crutches or a walker, he may prefer carrying items in a canvas, vinyl, or nylon *knapsack* strapped to his back. However, make sure he has good arm strength and balance before recommending a knapsack. Also, warn him not to attempt carrying heavy items in the knapsack.
• If none of these carrying aids seems adequate, remind your patient that he can have one custom made to fit his needs.

Selecting a reacher

If your patient's using crutches, a cane, a walker, or a wheelchair, he may want to reach an object beyond his grasp. In some cases, your patient may be able to ask someone to get the item for him. But, tell him that he can use a reacher to get the object himself.

Reachers come in a variety of sizes and styles, and are available at most medical supply stores. Three different models are shown here.

As you know, some reachers have magnetized tips for picking up small metal objects, such as safety pins. Others are equipped with hooked ends for picking up nonmetal objects, for example, sweaters, pens, or pencils.

Remind your patient that ordinary kitchen tongs or a bent metal clothes hanger can double as a reacher in some situations.

Finally, be sure to tell your patient to keep his reacher within easy access. He may want to hang it from his wheelchair or bedside table.

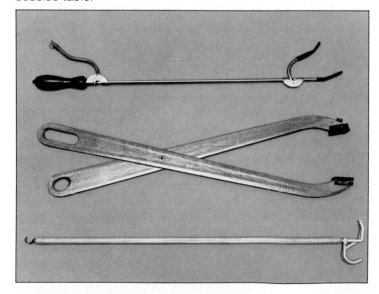

Environmental considerations

Questions and answers: How can your patient adapt his home to his needs?

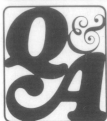

Are you helping your patient plan for his return home? If so, he may ask you how he can adapt his home to his needs. You'll want to answer any questions he has and offer possible solutions to his problems. To do so, familiarize yourself with the adaptive equipment on the market.

Remember: If your patient's weakness is temporary or changing, recommend he rent the equipment he'll need. Or, suggest he buy less expensive models because he'll use them for only a short time.

Here are answers to some questions your patient or his family may ask:

Patient's question: The walkway in front of my home is gravel. Will I be able to propel my wheelchair over it?
How to answer: Suggest your patient have the walkway paved or the gravel removed to create a smooth, level surface from the car to the door of his home. Or, if the patient spends a lot of time outdoors, suggest a wheelchair with pneumatic tires.

Patient's question: I must climb several steps to get into my home. How can I get up the steps with my wheelchair?
How to answer: If your patient is using a wheelchair and owns his home, suggest he have a ramp built over the steps, if possible.

But, he should make sure the ramp's incline is gradual, allowing a 1' (30.5 cm) length of ramp for each inch (2.54 cm) of elevation. The ramp should have a nonslip surface and at least one handrail that is about 32" (81 cm) high and extends at least 18" (46 cm) beyond the top and bottom steps. The ramp should have a flat platform 5' (1.5 m) square at the top (for turning), and at least a 6' (1.8 m) square clearance at the base.

If your patient can't install a ramp in his home, he may be able to go up and down the stairs in a sitting position, as described on pages 144 to 147. But, remind your patient that he'll need someone to transport his wheelchair, or keep a second wheelchair upstairs.

Suppose your patient can't go up the stairs this way either. Two people may have to carry him up the stairs, using a two-person lift (see pages 80 and 81).

Remember: If your patient will be using crutches or a cane to go up stairs, make sure there's a handrail for him to grasp on both sides of the stairs.

Patient's question: I have stairs inside my home. How can I go up and down these stairs with my wheelchair?
How to answer: Because your patient won't be able to build a ramp over the stairs inside his home, he'll use the sitting method to go up and down these stairs (see pages 144 to 147). Again, he'll need someone to carry his wheelchair.

Or, your patient may want to have an electric stair-climber installed. If he uses this device, he'll still need someone to transport his wheelchair up and down the steps, or suggest he keep a second chair upstairs.

☎ *Nursing tip:* If your patient's home has a bathroom downstairs, and he has an extra room available, suggest he convert one of the rooms on that level into a bedroom. By doing so, he'll eliminate having to go up and down stairs so frequently.

If your patient lives in an apartment and must climb many steps, recommend he move into a ground-floor apartment without stairs. Tell him he can contact your hospital's social service department for further assistance.

Patient's question: What width must doorways be to accommodate my wheelchair?
How to answer: Most wheelchairs are 25" (63.5 cm) wide, so doorways should be at least 27" (69 cm) wide. If the doorways in your patient's home aren't wide enough, suggest he have a wheelchair custom made to fit through the doorway, or obtain a wheelchair narrowing device. Or, if he owns his own home, suggest he remove the molding around the doorways to widen them. Recommend calling in a carpenter to widen the doorways only as a last resort.

Patient's question: My home has thick carpeting throughout. Can I use my wheelchair on it?
How to answer: Propelling a wheelchair over thick carpet (just as moving it over sand, grass, or soil) requires considerable arm strength. If your patient doesn't have strong arms, recommend he replace or remove the carpet.

A patient can use crutches, a cane, or a walker fairly easily on thick carpeting. However, rubber tips on these walking aids may catch in a shag carpet.

Hardwood, tile, or linoleum floors provide the best surface for a patient using a wheelchair or walking aid. But, remind your patient to avoid walking on slippery, waxed, or wet floors.

Caution: Warn your patient to remove small area rugs from his home. They increase the risk of accidents for a patient using a wheelchair or walking aid.

Patient's question: Should my bed at home be the same height as my wheelchair?
How to answer: If your patient will be using his wheelchair for a long period of time, he may want to get a bed the same height as his wheelchair seat. In most cases, he'll need to raise his bed about 4" (10 cm). Or, suggest your patient buy or rent a hospital bed with adjustable height.

Patient's question: What about the other furniture in my house? Will it create problems for me?
How to answer: If your patient is using a wheelchair or has difficulty getting out of a low seat, he should consider getting a raised toilet seat or a commode chair. Also, he may want to raise the cushion of his favorite armchair.

Recommend that your patient rearrange his furniture to create enough space to maneuver his wheelchair or walking aid. The standard wheelchair needs a space 60" x 60" (152 x 152 cm) in which to turn. A patient using a cane, crutches, or a walker needs a space at least 31" (79 cm) wide in which to walk.

Patient's question: Will I need to replace or add to the fixtures in my bathroom?
How to answer: If your patient has a shower stall, instead of a bathtub, suggest he obtain a shower chair.

In a bathtub, your patient can use a tub seat. If he has sensory loss in the lower portion of his body, make sure he fills the tub and checks the water temperature before getting in, so he doesn't burn himself.

For a patient with good hand strength, recommend a hand-held shower hose. But, again, remind him to test the water temperature first.

Recommend hanging mirrors, shelves, and towel bars at a lower level if your patient will be using a wheelchair. And, suggest handrails for bathroom and hallway walls if your patient has a walking aid.

Patient's question: I like to cook. Can I continue this activity from my wheelchair?
How to answer: In most kitchens, the counters, stoves, and cabinets are too high for a patient in a wheelchair. Your patient can use a reacher to remove objects from an overhead cabinet, but he won't be able to use a reacher to place a pot on the stove.

Suggest that your patient have his kitchen remodeled to meet his needs. For example, he can have the height of the counters reduced and obtain a lower range with an easy-to-reach control panel. (For more tips on how your patient can have his kitchen remodeled, contact your hospital's physical therapy department or the Easter Seal Society.)

If your patient will be using crutches, a cane, or a walker at home, he won't need his kitchen remodeled. But, he must find ways to free his hands so he can cook. Suggest he sit on a bar stool during meal preparation or use a walker with an attached seat.

Patient's question: I won't be able to get my wheelchair close to my kitchen sink because the legrests will hit the under-sink cabinet. How can I solve this problem?
How to answer: Recommend your patient empty the cabinet and remove its door. Although he may lose some storage space doing this, he'll gain the maneuverability he needs.

Caution: Are the water pipes below the sink exposed? If so, warn your patient about the possibility of burning his legs. A patient with paraplegia should have these pipes covered (not enclosed) so he isn't burned without realizing it.

Patient's question: I don't think I can afford the expense of having my home adapted in these ways.
How to answer: Refer your patient to the hospital's social service department or to another agency that can provide financial assistance. Depending on hospital policy, this referral may require a doctor's order.

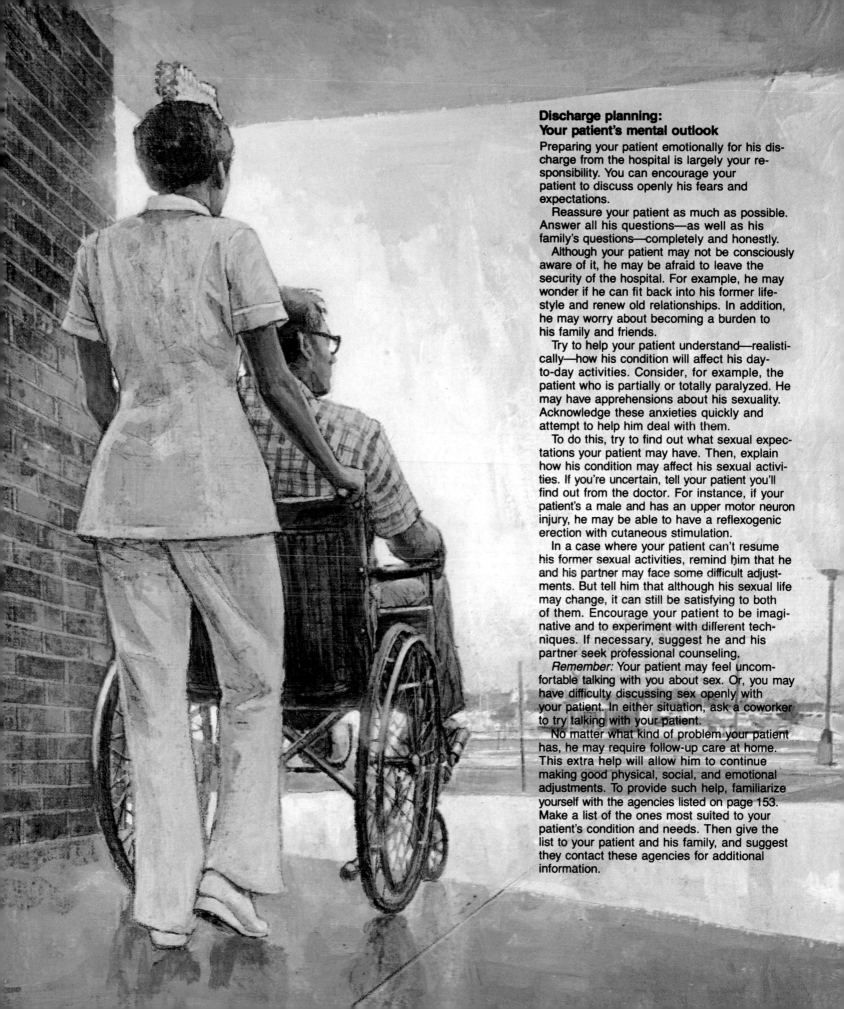

Discharge planning:
Your patient's mental outlook

Preparing your patient emotionally for his discharge from the hospital is largely your responsibility. You can encourage your patient to discuss openly his fears and expectations.

Reassure your patient as much as possible. Answer all his questions—as well as his family's questions—completely and honestly.

Although your patient may not be consciously aware of it, he may be afraid to leave the security of the hospital. For example, he may wonder if he can fit back into his former lifestyle and renew old relationships. In addition, he may worry about becoming a burden to his family and friends.

Try to help your patient understand—realistically—how his condition will affect his day-to-day activities. Consider, for example, the patient who is partially or totally paralyzed. He may have apprehensions about his sexuality. Acknowledge these anxieties quickly and attempt to help him deal with them.

To do this, try to find out what sexual expectations your patient may have. Then, explain how his condition may affect his sexual activities. If you're uncertain, tell your patient you'll find out from the doctor. For instance, if your patient's a male and has an upper motor neuron injury, he may be able to have a reflexogenic erection with cutaneous stimulation.

In a case where your patient can't resume his former sexual activities, remind him that he and his partner may face some difficult adjustments. But tell him that although his sexual life may change, it can still be satisfying to both of them. Encourage your patient to be imaginative and to experiment with different techniques. If necessary, suggest he and his partner seek professional counseling.

Remember: Your patient may feel uncomfortable talking with you about sex. Or, you may have difficulty discussing sex openly with your patient. In either situation, ask a coworker to try talking with your patient.

No matter what kind of problem your patient has, he may require follow-up care at home. This extra help will allow him to continue making good physical, social, and emotional adjustments. To provide such help, familiarize yourself with the agencies listed on page 153. Make a list of the ones most suited to your patient's condition and needs. Then give the list to your patient and his family, and suggest they contact these agencies for additional information.

Environmental considerations

Helping your patient adapt his home

You'll have to know some specific architectural information about your patient's home before you can suggest possible home adaptations. To obtain this information, ask your patient's family to complete and return a photocopy of the home assessment form on pages 154 and 155. Then, study the sample house shown here. It'll give you some home adaptation ideas you can suggest to your patient and his family.

Here's a detailed list of the adaptations we've shown at right:

In the living room
• low-pile carpet
• raised cushion on easy chair
• handrails along walls
• easy access to desk
• telephone on desk
• furniture arranged along walls for more moving space

In the kitchen
• floor kept dry, without excessive wax; no area rugs
• open cabinet areas under sink
• lowered counter space
• lowered storage space
• stove with easy-to-reach controls
• refrigerator door handle on right
• mirror angled over cooking surface
• easy-to-reach telephone
• adaptors hanging on a pegboard within reach

In the bedroom
• hospital-type bed with side rails and attached trapeze
• handrails along walls
• commode chair
• visual access to window from bed
• telephone placed on overbed table
• low-pile carpet

In the bathroom
• handrails along walls
• safety rails or grab bars around toilet and bathtub
• elevated toilet seat
• nonslip strips in bathtub
• hand-held shower head
• tub seat (chair)

In other areas
• ramp leading into house
• electric stair-climber
• smoke or heat detector on each floor
• fire extinguisher in kitchen and bedroom
• wide door frames
• handrails along all hallways
• fire escape from second story or bedroom

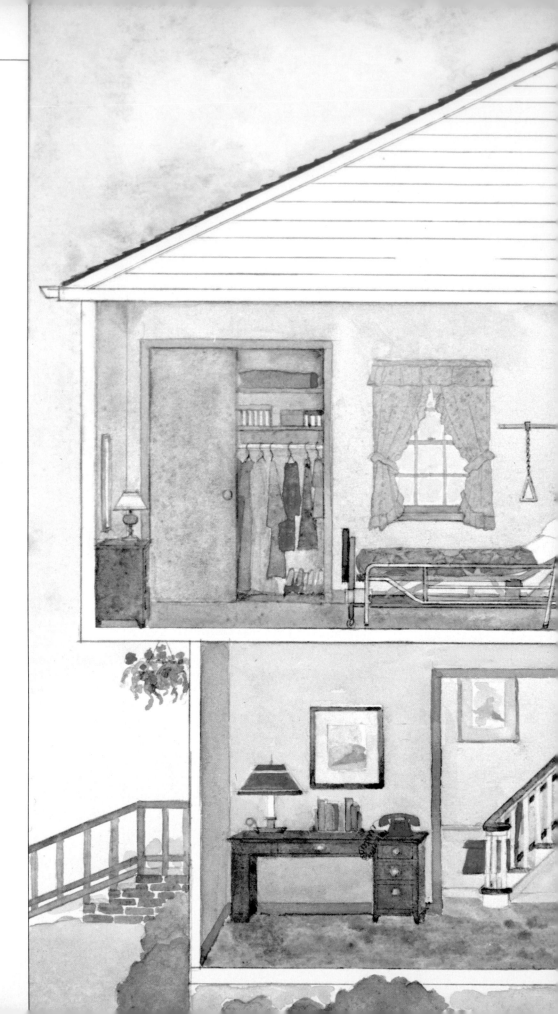

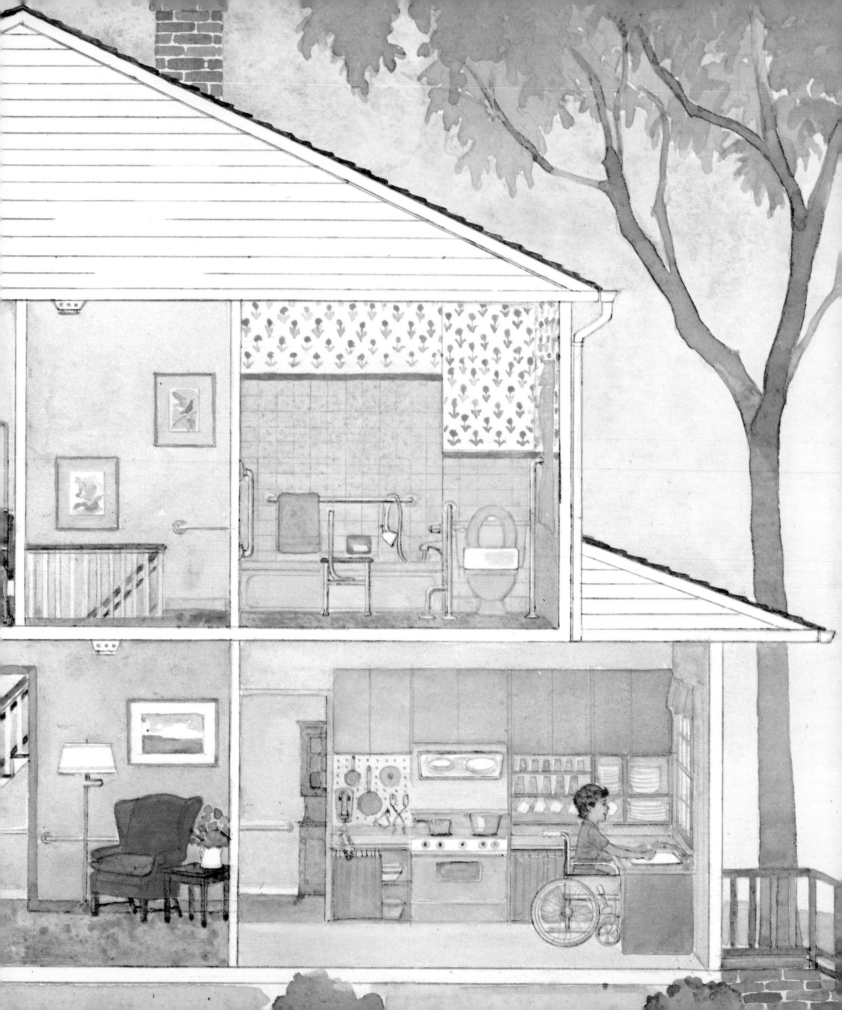

Environmental considerations

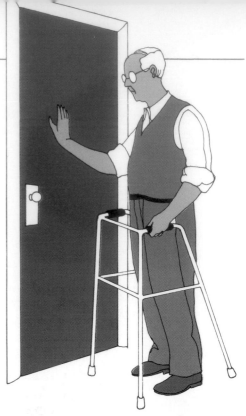

Special considerations: Some fire safety tips

On the last two pages, we've shown you some ways your patient can adapt his home for his comfort and needs. Now, we'll familiarize you with some fire safety considerations that are especially important for a patient with limited mobility.

As you know, if your patient's using crutches, a cane, a walker, or a wheelchair, he'll need extra time to vacate his home in an emergency. However, by reviewing some fire safety tips with your patient, you can help him save precious seconds—and his life.

Begin by asking your patient to list possible exits from his home. If his family's present, encourage them to be involved in the plan. But, remember, they may not always be home in an emergency. If your patient lives in an apartment, tell him to list all the fire escapes and stairways. But, warn him never to use an elevator as an emergency exit, because he could get trapped. Suggest practice fire drills, no matter where your patient lives.

Has your patient included a window as an emergency exit? If so, tell him to be sure he can open and close the window easily. Also, suggest he have the window screen removed. Or, have a push-out screen installed.

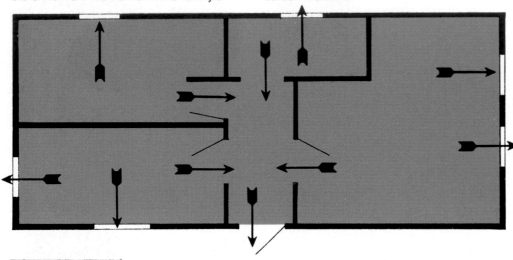

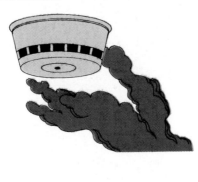

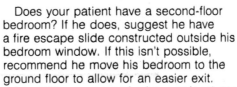

Does your patient have a second-floor bedroom? If he does, suggest he have a fire escape slide constructed outside his bedroom window. If this isn't possible, recommend he move his bedroom to the ground floor to allow for an easier exit.

In addition, suggest he have at least one smoke or heat detector installed outside his bedroom.

Note: We recommend one smoke or heat detector per floor. Your patient should also keep fire extinguishers in his bedroom and kitchen.

Here are some safety considerations to review with your patient and his family:
• Tell your patient to sleep with his bedroom door closed. If he suspects a fire, instruct him to touch his bedroom door before opening it. Warn him *never* to open a door that feels hot. Instead, he should place a rolled sheet or blanket under the door to prevent smoke from circulating into his bedroom. Then, tell him to choose an alternate exit, for example, a window.
• In case of fire, tell your patient to leave his home as quickly as possible. But, suggest he keep a list of emergency telephone numbers next to a telephone on a bedside table, in case he should become trapped in his bedroom.

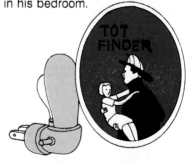

• Recommend he have night lights installed around the inside of his home. By doing this, he can safely find his way to an exit in an emergency.

Finally, advise your patient and his family to contact their local fire department. In most cases, a representative can visit their home and make suggestions for possible safety adaptations. He can supply emergency window decals and teach the patient and his family various lifts and evacuation techniques to make an emergency exit fast and efficient.

Agencies

For additional help and information:

Action
806 Connecticut Ave., N.W.
Washington, D.C. 20525

American Association of Retired Persons
National Headquarters
1909 K St., N.W.
Washington, D.C. 20049

American Cancer Society, Inc. National Office
777 Third Ave.
New York, N.Y. 10017

American Diabetes Association, Inc.
600 Fifth Ave.
New York, N.Y. 10020

American Dietetic Association
430 North Michigan Ave.
Chicago, Ill. 60611

American Foundation for the Blind
15 West 16th St.
New York, N.Y. 10011

American Home Economics Association
2010 Massachusetts Ave., N.W.
Washington, D.C. 20036

American Lung Association
1740 Broadway
New York, N.Y. 10019

American Medical Association
535 N. Dearborn St.
Chicago, Ill. 60610

American Occupational Therapy Association, Inc.
1383 Piccard Dr., Suite 300
Rockville, Md. 20850

American Physical Therapy Association

1156 15th St., N.W.
Washington, D.C. 20006

Arthritis Foundation
Lenox P.O. Box 18888
Atlanta, Ga. 30326

Disabled Veterans of America
P.O. Box 4301
Cincinnati, Ohio 45201

Federation of the Handicapped
211 West 14th St.
New York, N.Y. 10011

Institute of Rehabilitation Medicine
New York University
Medical Center
400 East 34th St.
New York, N.Y. 10016

International Federation on Aging
1909 K St., N.W.
Washington, D.C. 20049

Library of Congress National Library Service for the Blind and Physically Handicapped
Washington, D.C. 20542

March of Dimes Birth Defects Foundation
1275 Mamaroneck Ave.
White Plains, N.Y. 10605

Medic Alert Foundation International
P.O. Box 1009
Turlock, Calif. 95380

Muscular Dystrophy Association
810 Seventh Ave.
New York, N.Y. 10019

National Association for the Physically Handicapped
Meetinghouse Rd.
Merrimack, N.H. 03054

National Association of Rehabilitation Facilities
5530 Wisconsin Ave.
Suite 955
Washington, D.C. 20015

National Association of Social Workers
600 Southern Building
15th and H Streets, N.W.
Washington, D.C. 20005

National Center for Citizen Involvement
1214 16th St., N.W.
Washington, D.C. 20036

National Council of Senior Citizens
1511 K St., N.W.
Washington, D.C. 20005

National Council on the Aging
1828 L St., N.W.
Washington, D.C. 20036

National Easter Seal Society
2023 West Ogden Ave.
Chicago, Ill. 60612

National HomeCaring Council
67 Irving Pl.
New York, N.Y. 10003

National Institute of Arthritis and Metabolic Diseases
Bethesda, Md. 20205

National League for Nursing
10 Columbus Circle
New York, N.Y. 10019

National Rehabilitation Association
633 Washington St.
Alexandria, Va. 22314

National Society to Prevent Blindness
79 Madison Ave.
New York, N.Y. 10016

President's Committee on Employment of the Handicapped
Washington, D.C. 20210

Public Affairs Pamphlets
381 Park Ave. South
New York, N.Y. 10016

Senior Citizen Service Organizations
(Check local telephone directory)

Sister Kenny Institute
Publications-Audiovisuals Office
2727 Chicago Ave.
Minneapolis, Minn. 55407

Superintendent of Documents
U.S. Government Printing Office
Washington, D.C. 20402

United Cerebral Palsy Association
66 East 34th St.
New York, N.Y. 10016

U.S. Department of Health, Education, and Welfare Office of Information National Heart, Lung, and Blood Institute
Bethesda, Md. 20205

Urban Mass Transit Transportation Administration
Office of Public Affairs
400 7th St., S.W.
Washington, D.C. 20590

Visiting Nurse Association
(Check local telephone directory)

Vocational Guidance and Rehabilitation Services
2239 East 55th St.
Cleveland, Ohio 44103

Environmental considerations

HOME ASSESSMENT FORM

NAME: DATE:

TYPE OF HOME:

☐ Two-story   ☐ Ranch

☐ Split-level   ☐ Apartment

For apartment dweller:

☐ What floor   ☐ Elevator
                     available

If steps are present in the house:

Number

Width

Height

Depth

Handrails

☐ Right side   ☐ Both

☐ Left side

ENTRANCES:

How many and location of each

If steps are present outside the house:

Number

Width

Depth

Height

Clearance around base of steps:

BATHROOM:

How many

Location

Room dimensions

Door width

☐ Tub

☐ Shower

☐ Sink

Height from floor

Toilet seat height

Draw a floor plan, including location of wall studs, windows, and doorway.

KITCHEN:

Counter height

Stove height, and location of controls

Room dimensions

Door width

Draw a floor plan, including location of appliances, counter, windows and doorways.

BEDROOM:

On which floor is bedroom located.

Room dimensions

Door width

Bed height

Draw a floor plan including
location of windows, closets, and
doorways.

OTHER ROOM:

Room

Dimensions

Doorway width

Additional comments:

Draw a floor plan of each
additional room, including
windows, doorways and closets.

OTHER ROOM:

Room

Dimensions

Doorway width

Additional comments:

Selected references

Books

Basmajian, John V. THERAPEUTIC EXERCISE, 3rd ed. Baltimore: Williams & Wilkins Co., 1978.

Bilger, Annetta, and Ellen Greene, eds. WINTERS' PROTECTIVE BODY MECHANICS. New York: Springer Publishing Co., 1973.

Boroch, Rose. ELEMENTS OF REHABILITATION IN NURSING: AN INTRODUCTION. St. Louis: C.V. Mosby Co., 1976.

Buchwald, Edith. PHYSICAL REHABILITATION FOR DAILY LIVING. New York: McGraw-Hill Book Co., 1952.

Christopherson, Victor A., et al. REHABILITATION NURSING: PERSPECTIVES AND APPLICATIONS. New York: McGraw-Hill Book Co., 1974.

COPING WITH NEUROLOGIC PROBLEMS PROFICIENTLY. *Nursing* Skillbook® Series. Horsham, Pa.: Intermed Communications, Inc., 1979.

DuGas, Beverly W. KOZIER-DUGAS' INTRODUCTION TO PATIENT CARE, 2nd ed. Philadelphia: W.B. Saunders Co., 1972.

Eldridge, Priscilla B. CARING FOR THE DISABLED PATIENT: AN ILLUSTRATED GUIDE. Oradell, N.J.: Medical Economics Co., 1978.

Farrell, Jane. ILLUSTRATED GUIDE TO ORTHOPEDIC NURSING. Philadelphia: J.B. Lippincott Co., 1977.

Flaherty, Patricia T., and Sandra J. Jurkovich. TRANSFERS FOR PATIENTS WITH ACUTE AND CHRONIC CONDITIONS. Minneapolis: Sister Kenny Institute, 1970.

Ford, Jack R., and Bridget Duckworth. PHYSICAL MANAGEMENT FOR THE QUADRIPLEGIC. Philadelphia: F.A. Davis Co., 1974.

Gilbert, Arlene E. YOU CAN DO IT FROM A WHEELCHAIR. New Rochelle, N.Y.: Arlington House Publishers, 1974.

Hardy, Alan G., and Reginald Elson. PRACTICAL MANAGEMENT OF SPINAL INJURY FOR NURSES, 2nd ed. London: Churchill Livingstone, Inc., 1976.

Hirschberg, Gerald G., et al. REHABILITATION: A MANUAL FOR THE CARE OF THE DISABLED AND ELDERLY, 2nd ed. Philadelphia: J.B. Lippincott Co., 1976.

Lowman, Edward, and Judith Klinger. AIDS TO INDEPENDENT LIVING: SELF-HELP FOR THE HANDICAPPED. New York: McGraw-Hill Book Co., 1969.

MEALTIME MANUAL FOR PEOPLE WITH DISABILITIES AND THE AGING. Camden, N.J.: Campbell Soup Co., 1978.

Mital, Mohinder A., and Donald S. Pierce. AMPUTEES AND THEIR PROSTHESES. Boston: Little, Brown & Co., 1971.

Murray, Rosemary, and Jean Kijek. CURRENT PERSPECTIVES IN REHABILITATION NURSING. St. Louis: C.V. Mosby Co., 1979.

O'Brien, Mary T., and Phyllis J. Pallett. TOTAL CARE OF THE STROKE PATIENT. Boston: Little, Brown & Co., 1978.

Rantz, Marilyn J., and Donald Courtial. LIFTING, MOVING, AND TRANSFERRING PATIENTS: A MANUAL. St. Louis: C.V. Mosby Co., 1977.

Rusk, Howard A., ed. REHABILITATION MEDICINE. St. Louis: C.V. Mosby Co., 1977.

SAFETY AND HANDLING OF WHEELCHAIRS. Los Angeles: Everest & Jennings, Inc., 1976.

Sorenson, Lois, and Patricia G. Ulrich. AMBULATION GUIDE FOR NURSES. Minneapolis: Sister Kenny Institute, 1977.

Stryker, Ruth. REHABILITATIVE ASPECTS OF ACUTE AND CHRONIC NURSING CARE, 2nd ed. Philadelphia: W.B. Saunders Co., 1977.

Talbot, Dianne. PRINCIPLES OF THERAPEUTIC POSITIONING: A GUIDE FOR NURSING ACTION. Minneapolis: Sister Kenny Institute, 1978.

Toohey, Patricia, and Corrine W. Larson. RANGE OF MOTION EXERCISE: KEY TO JOINT MOBILITY. Minneapolis: Sister Kenny Institute, 1977.

Periodicals

Bame, Black Kathleen. *Halo Traction,* AMERICAN JOURNAL OF NURSING. 69:1933-37, September 1969.

Caring for the Totally Dependent Patient: Some Traps—Some Guidelines, NURSING76. 6:38-43, July 1976.

Drapeau, Janine. *Getting Back into Good Posture: How to Erase Your Lumbar Aches,* NURSING75. 5:63-5, September 1975.

Ford, Jack R., and Bridget Duckworth. *Moving a Patient Safely, Comfortably: Part 1, Patient Positioning,* NURSING76. 6:27-36, January 1976; *Part 2, Transferring,* NURSING76. 6:58-65, February 1976.

Hirschberg, Gerald, et al. *Promoting Patient Mobility and Preventing Secondary Disabilities,* NURSING77. 7:42-7, May 1977.

How to Negotiate the Ups and Downs, Ins and Outs of Body Alignment, NURSING74. 4:46-51, October 1974.

Long, Barbara C., and Patricia S. Buergin. *The Pivot Transfer,* AMERICAN JOURNAL OF NURSING. 7:980-982, June 1977.

Redman, Barbara K. *Patient Education as a Function of Nursing Practice,* NURSING CLINICS OF NORTH AMERICA. 6:573-80, December 1971.

Rozen, Raphael. *Car Independence for Patients with Triplegia,* ARCHIVES OF PHYSICAL MEDICINE AND REHABILITATION. 52:80, February 1971.

Rusk, Howard. *Rehabilitation Belongs in the General Hospital,* AMERICAN JOURNAL OF NURSING. 62:62-3, September 1962.

Acknowledgements

Index

**We'd like to thank
the following people
and companies
for their help
with this PHOTOBOOK:**

AACOMED HOSPITAL EQUIPMENT & SUPPLIES
Philadelphia, Pa.
Harry Weiler, Manager

ACCURATE MEDICAL SERVICE
Willow Grove, Pa.
Steve Wharton, Manager

ACTIVEaid, INC.
Redwood Falls, Minn.
Charles H. Nearing, Vice-President

ALL ORTHOPEDIC APPLIANCES (AOA)
Greenwood, S.C.
George Rosselle, Product Manager

CLINIC SHOEMAKERS
Aurora, Mo.

GUARDIAN PRODUCTS CO., INC.
North Hollywood, Calif.

HEALTHCO, INC.
Reading, Pa.
Al Szymborski, CMR

LUMEX, INC.
Bay Shore, N.Y.
William Kelly,
Sales Administrator

J.T. POSEY CO.
Arcadia, Calif.

FRED SAMMONS, INC.
Brookfield, Ill.

SCIMEDICS, INC.
Anaheim, Calif.
Margaret G. Rogers, President
John E. Rogers, MS, Consultant

SPAN-AMERICA, INC.
Greenville, S.C.
Donald C. Spann, President

TRANS-AID CORP.
Carson, Calif.

Also the staffs of:
MAGEE MEMORIAL REHABILITATION CENTER
Philadelphia, Pa.

QUAKERTOWN HOSPITAL
Quakertown, Pa.

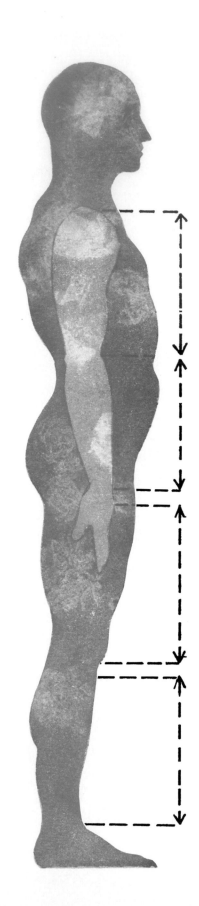

A

Abduction pillow. See *Positioning aids*.
Agencies, for additional help, 153
Air mattress. See *Mattresses*.
Amputation, leg
  bandaging
    above the knee, 62-63
    below the knee, 64-65
  patient preparation, 62
  plaster cast, care of, 66
  strengthening exercises, 66-68
Arm splint. See *Positioning aids*.
Assessment, mental and physical, 11

B

Bandaging
  above-the-knee amputation, 62-63
  below-the knee amputation, 64-65
Bed cradle. See *Positioning aids*.
Body mechanics
  how to improve, 13-17
  how to move an object, 16-17
  how to reach properly, 16-17
Bridging technique, 30

C

Canes
  getting in and out of a chair, 120-121
  going up and down stairs, 122-123
  how to choose
    broad-based, 116
    regular, 117
    T-handle and J-line, 117
  walking, 118-120
Carrying devices, 147
Car transfers
  using mechanical lifter, 94-96
  using stand-pivot, 84-85
  using transfer board, 100-101
Commode chair, 73
Cradle boot. See *Positioning aids*.
Crutches
  coping with falls, 142-143
  picking up an item from the floor, 138
  proper fit, 104
Crutches, canes, and walkers
  gait selection guidelines, 104
  helpful hints, 104
  reachers, 147
Crutch-walking

four-point gait, 106-107
gait selection guidelines, 104
getting in and out of a chair,
    112-113
three-point gait (non-
    weight–bearing), 108-109
three-point-and-one gait
    (partial-weight–bearing),
    110-111
two-point gait, 105
up and down stairs, 114-115

D

Discharge planning
    agencies for additional help,
        153
    fire safety, 152
    home adaptations, 150-151
    mental outlook, 149
    questions and answers, 148
Drawsheet, moving a patient
    from back to side-lying posi-
        tion, 32-33
    from side-lying to prone, 38
    logroll, 36-37
    up in bed, 27

E

Egg crate mattress. See *Mat-
    tresses.*
Elbow protector. See *Positioning
    aids.*

F

Finger contraction cushion. See
    Positioning aids.
Fire safety, 152
Flotation pad mattress. See
    Mattresses.
Footboard. See *Positioning aids.*
Footdrop stop. See *Positioning
    aids.*
Foot-guard. See *Positioning aids.*
Four-point gait
    crutches, 106-107
    reciprocal walkers, 126-127

G

Goal setting
    how to help your patient set
        short- or long-term goals,
        12
    nurses' role, 12

H

Halo traction, transferring a
    patient with, 91
Hand roll. See *Positioning aids.*
Hazards of immobility. See
    Mobility hazards.
Heel protector. See *Positioning
    aids.*
Home assessment form, 154-155
Home care aids
    how to do isometric exercises,
        61
    how to perform a forward-
        backward sitting transfer,
        89
    how to strengthen your mus-
        cles after a mastectomy,
        69

I

Isometric exercises, 60-61

L

Leg-dangling position, how to
    place patient in, 42-43
Leg splint. See *Positioning aids.*
Logrolling a spinal-injured
    patient, 35 37

M

Mastectomy, strengthening
    exercises after, 68-69
Mattresses
    air, 20
    egg crate, 21
    flotation pad, 21
    sheepskin, 21
    water, 20
Mechanical lifter
    car transfer, 94-96
    description, 72-73
    moving patient from bed to
        wheelchair, 92-93
Mini-assessment, Range of
    motion (ROM): How to
    choose your patient's exer-
    cise program, 46
Mobility hazards, how to detect
    cardiovascular, 18
    gastrointestinal, 19
    genitourinary, 19
    integumentary, 18
    muscular, 18
    neurologic, 19
    respiratory, 19
    skeletal, 19

N

Non-weight–bearing gait. See
    Three-point gait.

P

Partial-weight–bearing gait. See
    Three-point-and-one gait.
Patient roller board. See *Roller
    board.*
Positioning. See *Turning and
    positioning.*
Positioning aids
    abduction pillow, 22
    arm splint, 25
    bed cradle, 25
    cradle boot, 22
    drawsheet, 27, 32-33, 36-37,
        38
    elbow protector, 25
    finger contracture cushion, 24
    footboard, 23
    footdrop stop, 23
    foot-guard, 24
    hand roll, 22
    heel protector, 24
    leg splint, 25
    pillow, 22
    prone pillow, 23
    trochanter roll, 23
    turn and hold sheet, 24
Posture. See *Body mechanics.*
Pressure relief aids
    air mattress, 20
    egg crate mattress, 21
    flotation pad mattress, 21
    sheepskin, 21
    water mattress, 20
Prone pillow. See *Positioning
    aids.*
Prone position, how to place
    patient in, 38-40

R

Range of motion
    ankles, 59
    basic terms, 46
    choosing an exercise program,
        46
    elbows, 51
    feet, 60
    fingers, 53
    forearms, 51
    hands, 53
    hips, 55-57
    knees, 58
    neck, 47
    passive, 46
    shoulders, 48-50
    thumbs, 54
    toes, 60

Index

wrists, 52
Reachers, 147
Roller board, how to use, 90-91

S

Sheepskin. See *Pressure relief aids.*
Shower seat, 73
Side-lying position, how to place patient in, 31-35
Skin care schedule. See *Turning and positioning.*
Strengthening exercises
　after a leg amputation, 66-68
　isometric exercises, 60-61
　postmastectomy, 68-69
　range of motion, 46-60
Stretcher, 74
Supine position, how to support patient in, 29-30

T

Three-point gait, how to teach
　patient on crutches, 108-109
　patient with stationary walker, 126-127
Three-point-and-one gait, how to teach
　patient on crutches, 110-111
　patient with walker, 126-127
Traction, how to move a patient in
　Buck's traction, 40-41
　halo traction, 91
Transfer belt, 75
Transfer board
　description, 74
　moving patient with, 98-99
　performing car transfer, 100-101
　suggestions for use, 97
　teaching patient how to use, 97
Transfer equipment
　commode chair, 73
　mechanical lifter, 72-73
　patient roller board, 74
　shower seat, 73
　stretcher, 74
　transfer belt, 75
　transfer board, 74
　tub seat, 72-73
Transfer techniques
　bed to stretcher, 78-79
　evaluating, 75
　mechanical lifter. See *Mechanical lifter.*
　patient in halo traction, 91
　selecting, 72
　sitting, forward-backward, 89
　sitting, from bed to wheelchair, 88

sitting, with transfer board
　into a car, 100-101
　moving patient, 98-99
　teaching patient, 97
　standing, bed to wheelchair, 86-87
　stand-pivot
　　into car, 84-85
　　into wheelchair, 82-83
　three-person lift, 76-77
　two-person lift, 80-81
　with patient roller board, 90-91
Trochanter roll. See *Positioning aids.*
Tub seat, 72-73
Turn and hold sheet. See *Positioning aids.*
Turning and positioning
　bridging technique, 30
　leg-dangling position, 42-43
　logrolling a spinal-injured patient, 35-37
　moving a patient in traction, 40-41
　moving a patient up in bed, 26-27
　positioning and skin care schedule, 28
　positioning in a chair, 44-45
　prone position, 38-40
　side-lying position, 31-35
　supine position, 29-30
Two-point gait, how to teach
　patient on crutches, 105
　patient with reciprocal walker, 125

W

Walkers
　coping with falls, 143
　getting in and out of a chair, 128
　how to select, 124-125
　picking up an item from the floor, 139
　reciprocal
　　four-point gait, 126-127
　　two-point gait, 125
　stationary
　　three-point gait (non-weight–bearing), 126-127
　　three-point-and-one gait (partial-weight–bearing), 126-127
Walking belt. See *Transfer belt.*
Water mattress. See *Mattresses.*
Wheelchairs
　carrying devices, 147
　coping with falls, 140-141
　going up and down stairs, 144-147
　parts and function, 130-132
　picking up an item from the floor, 136-137
　power-driven, 133
　selection, 129
　selection by condition, 133

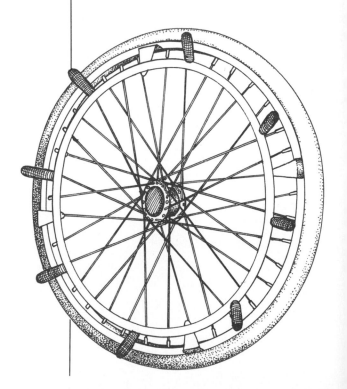